MW00512618

KETO DESSERTS COOKBOOK 2021

© Copyright 2021 All rights reserved.

This document is geared towards providing exact and reliable information with regards to the topic and issue covered. The publication is sold with the idea that the publisher is not required to render accounting, officially permitted, or otherwise, qualified services. If advice is necessary, legal or professional, a practiced individual in the profession should be ordered.

- From a Declaration of Principles which was accepted and approved equally by a Committee of the American Bar Association and a Committee of Publishers and Associations.

In no way is it legal to reproduce, duplicate, or transmit any part of this document in either electronic means or in printed format. Recording of this publication is strictly prohibited and any storage of this document is not allowed unless with written permission from the publisher. All rights reserved.

The information provided herein is stated to be truthful and consistent, in that any liability, in terms of inattention or otherwise, by any usage or abuse of any policies, processes, or directions contained within is the solitary and utter responsibility of the recipient reader. Under no circumstances will any legal responsibility or blame be held against the publisher for any reparation, damages, or monetary loss due to the information herein, either directly or indirectly.

Respective authors own all copyrights not held by the publisher.

The information herein is offered for informational purposes solely, and is universal as so. The presentation of the information is without contract or any type of guarantee assurance.
The trademarks that are used are without any consent, and the publication of the trademark is without permission or backing by the trademark owner. All trademarks and brands within this book are for clarifying purposes only and are the owned by the owners themselves, not affiliated with this document

Table of contents

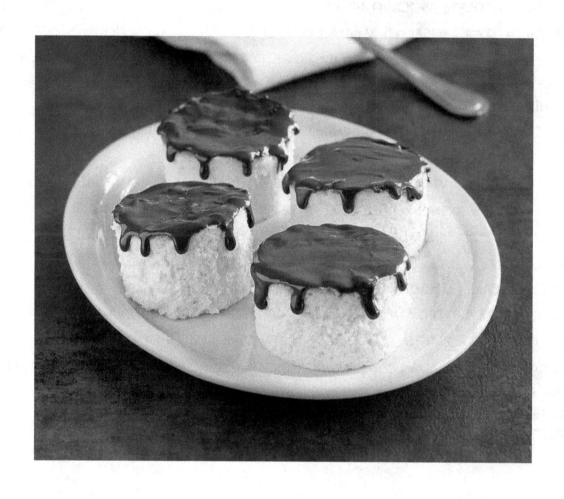

KETOGENIC DIET IN GENERAL

Essentially every health and fitness devotee and yo-yo dieter has found out about the ketogenic diet. It was initially evolved under clinical supervision for kids with epilepsy and another neurological issue. Notwithstanding, it has since taken the remainder of the world by storm absent a lot of disarray and debate.

All in all, what is the keto diet and its numerous health benefits?

To start, the human body has a chain of command for favored wellsprings of energy, with starches at the top. Fats come straightaway, and afterward at last proteins. In any case, one's present health and purpose behind utilizing a ketogenic diet for the most part direct the amount of each macronutrient is devoured.

The first and most significant idea is devouring a set number of carbs every day. The sum will, as a rule, be 25g or less to constrain the body into a state called "ketosis."

WHAT IS KETO DIET

The Ketogenic Diet is an uncommon diet high in fat, low in starches and moderate in protein, deliberately controlled. "Ketogenic" implies that a synthetic substance, called ketones, is delivered in the body (keto = ketones, beginning = creation).

The perfect Ketogenic Diet called the "long-chain triglyceride diet," gives 3 to 4 grams of fat for each gram of starch and protein. The "proportion" in the Ketogenic Diet is the proportion of fat for every gram of starch and protein joined. The kind of fat source foods of the Ketogenic Diet is margarine, cream or cream, mayonnaise, and oils.

Albeit the two starches and proteins in the diet are confined, it is basic to give enough measures of protein. It is likewise basic to set up the Ketogenic Diet painstakingly regulated by a Nutritionist, who observed the nutrition of the youngsters.

How Does The Keto Diet Work? How Does The Keto Diet Work?

Generally, the body utilizes starches (sugar, bread, or pasta) as its fuel, yet in the Ketogenic Diet, the fat turns into the essential fuel. Ketones are one of the potential instruments of activity of the diet. There are various speculations, for example, the adjustment of glucose, adenosine, polyunsaturated unsaturated fats, and then some.

For Whom Is The Keto Diet Appropriate?

It is recommended for youngsters with seizures that are hard-headed to treatment. That is, they don't react to a few diverse anticonvulsant prescriptions. They have been utilized first in quite a while. Be that as it may, it is especially recommended for kids with Lennox-Gastaut disorder.

It is additionally reasonable for particular sorts of seizures or epileptic disorders, being valuable for myoclonic epilepsy of youth (Dravet disorder), asthmatic myoclonic epilepsy (Doose disorder), puerile fits (West disorder), mitochondrial abandons, Tuberous sclerosis complex (TSC), Rett disorder. Furthermore, for the GLUT 1 insufficiency disorder (GLUT1 DS) and pyruvate dehydrogenase inadequacy (PDH).

How To Start The Keto Diet?

Commonly this diet is started in the clinic. The kid routinely starts with a quick or limited quantity of the food (aside from water) and under exacting clinical supervision for 24 hours. The principle motivation to enter them in many focuses is to screen any expansion in seizures with diet, treat hypoglycemia or acidosis, screen and improve resistance, guarantee that all drugs are liberated from starches, and teach the family to keep up the diet at home.

Does The Ketogenic Diet Work?

Around half of the kids who start the diet have at any rate a half decrease in the number of seizures, and other youngsters (10-15%) are liberated from seizures. Be that as it may, not all kids have more noteworthy control of the emergency, and some have different benefits, for example, being progressively alert, mindful, and with a superior reaction.

How To Monitor The Diet?

Pee test strips are utilized to screen the creation of ketones in the pee, delivered by the diet. Likewise, at regular intervals or thereabouts, other lab tests are performed to screen electrolytes, kidney work, liver capacity, carnitine, selenium, and others.

The Side Effects Of The Diet

The individual who begins the ketogenic diet may feel lethargic for a couple of days in the wake of beginning the diet. Opposite reactions that may happen incorporate kidney stones, high serum cholesterol levels, heaving, obstruction, poor development or weight increase, bone cracks, and that are only the tip of the iceberg.

TYPES OF KETOGENIC DIET

"Diet" signifies various things to various individuals. It can mean the sorts of foods an individual routinely eats. Moreover, it can mean an extraordinary course of food/food limitations either for weight reduction or clinical purposes.

Be that as it may, in the keto-world, diet implies both.

The ketogenic diet can be either a perpetual method for eating or a transitory health improvement plan. In any case, every individual's needs and objectives for utilizing this diet ought to be considered throughout the whole procedure.

STANDARD KETOGENIC DIET (SKD)

The proportion for the SKD rendition is regularly 5% carbs, 75% fat, and 20% protein. The numbers for fat and protein may move a bit. Be that as it may, generally, fat is a tremendous piece of the diet and caloric admission.

This very well known form uses this simple idea: basically remain at or underneath carb utmost to stay in ketosis.

HIGH PROTEIN KETOGENIC DIET

Right now, it is accomplished similarly as in the standard ketogenic diet. An ordinary macronutrient proportion may look like 55-60% fat, 35-40% protein, and still 5% carbs. Similarly, as with the SKD, one must stay at or underneath as far as possible for ketosis to do something amazing.

TARGETED KETOGENIC DIET (TKD)

Have you ever known about carb-stacking before an exercise? This is the principle thought with the focus on a ketogenic diet.

In this way, around 30-an hour prior to work out, eat somewhere in the range of 25-50g of effectively edible carbs. The genuine number will rely upon the person's needs and the sort of exercise to be performed.

The better kind of carbs for this keto rendition is glucose-based food. The body utilizes glucose-based food more proficiently than fructose-based food. To explain, glucose-based food is generally scorched totally without tossing the body out of ketosis.

At last, post-exercise meals ought to incorporate a lot of protein and less fat. In the typical keto circumstance, fat is supported. Nonetheless, for muscle recuperation and supplement retention, protein is a superior decision for the focus on the ketogenic diet.

CYCLICAL KETOGENIC DIET (CKD)

This one sounds weird, thinking about what we've been realizing. CKD is for weight lifters and competitors who wish to manufacture fit bulk and still boost fat misfortune.

Right now, keep a standard keto diet for five days. At that point, you cycle into the two-day period of carb-stacking.

As far as possible on the first carb-stacking day will be 50g. On the second carb-stacking day, the carb tally will be somewhere in the range of 400-600g. The reason is to stack up on carbs, so the body is appropriately energized for the following five days of tiring exercises.

Significantly, CKD carb stacking ought not to be utilized as a "cheat day" for those utilizing the standard ketogenic diet. This methodology is appropriate just for incredibly dynamic people.

RESTRICTED KETOGENIC DIET

Right now, both carbs and calories are restricted. Clinical experts, for the most part, direct this rendition. This form might be valuable in malignant growth treatment. In light of studies, disease cells can't utilize ketones for energy and actually can starve to death.

Likewise, with any diet routine or way of life change, you should look for the guidance of a proper clinical expert before starting. Such experts will think about the individual's clinical history and current condition of health, just as individual needs and objectives.

HEALTH BENEFITS OF THE KETO DIET

Individuals most normally partner the ketogenic diet with fast weight reduction. In any case, that is not where it got its beginning. Also, it's absolutely not the stopping point undoubtedly.

There's no denying that weight reduction alone guides in the advancement of by and large health. What's more, with weight reduction comes a large number of other cardiovascular and stomach related enhancements.

Notwithstanding, the rundown doesn't verge on halting there. We should take a gander at some different circumstances where this inconceivable method for eating has a constructive outcome.

EPILEPTIC SEIZURES

Initially, clinical experts built up the ketogenic diet to treat epilepsy in youngsters impervious to different prescriptions. In a 1920s report, Dr. Russell Wilder saw a 90% abatement in seizures in around 30% of subjects.

As one would expect, there was a huge drop in the number of patients staying in the examination. In any case, the outcomes were predictable with the rest of the subjects at the 3-month, half-year, and one-year interims.

Later information has discovered a half decrease in seizures in an assessment of very nearly 20 examinations with 1084 patients. Both with and without the utilization of anticonvulsant prescriptions, the ketogenic diet has been compelling in seizure decrease.

Intellectual prowess

In light of the extraordinary outcomes in epilepsy patients, more research has been in progress. Reassuringly, it is indicating promising outcomes in the treatment of Alzheimer's Disease and Parkinson's Disease. The investigations demonstrate expanded insight and upgraded memory.

Essentially, fit as a fiddle, people notice more noteworthy mental lucidity, expanded capacity to center, just as better headache control. The "why" isn't totally clear now.

CORONARY ILLNESS PREVENTION

Almost certainly, a large portion of us understands that weight reduction assists lower with blooding pressure. Furthermore, cholesterol levels additionally improve from along these lines of eating. The ketogenic diet advances a high-fat (healthy fat) routine with restricted sugars. This brings down triglycerides and expands HDLs (great cholesterol).

This appears to be insane from the start since everyone lets us know "fat" is terrible. What's more, specialists have been instructing patients for a considerable length of time to eat a low-fat, heart-healthy diet. In any case, in opposition to that hypothesis, starches, not fat, are really a huge main impetus behind expanded triglycerides.

POLYCYSTIC OVARY SYNDROME

Polycystic ovary disorder accompanies fluctuated side effects. These incorporate skin break out, state of mind swings, barrenness, exhaustion, skin labels, and hair development on the chest, face, back, and toes. It likewise causes excruciating and sporadic menstrual cycles. Moreover, most of those influenced by PCOS experience weight put on or issues shedding pounds.

In what manner can the ketogenic diet help PCOS? It's all hormonal. Expanded measures of the hormones insulin and androgen are the necessary team for a PCOS finding.

With the ketogenic diet, glucose levels go down as ketone levels go up. Lower glucose levels mean lower insulin levels. Thus, this implies the ovaries have no compelling reason to deliver more androgens, the male hormone. The outcome is the decrease or annihilation of PCOS indications, including fruitlessness. Gotta love that!

DIMINISHED INFLAMMATION ISSUES.

This classification incorporates joint inflammation, bad-tempered gut disorder (IBS), skin break out, and other skin issues. Fortunately for individuals with these issues, the ketogenic diet is essentially calming.

There are various kinds of ketones present in a nutritional ketosis state. One of these smothers an irritation particle usually found in incendiary procedures. In light of this marvelous connection between the ketogenic diet and incendiary help, more research is prospective.

GASTROINTESTINAL PROBLEMS

There is incredible news for people with gastrointestinal issues, for example, gas, swelling, indigestion, and heartburn. Grains, especially wheat, rye, and grain, are a food stick helping the grain hold its shape. The ketogenic diet is a without grain method for eating. In this way, these side effects ought to reduce or totally decrease just by following the plan.

Another guilty party for stomach and stomach related problems is sugary foods. Since the ketogenic diet's primary idea is low-carb, sugars won't be an issue for the belly either.

KETO DESSERTS

Aside from being ideal for a keto diet, practically the entirety of the desserts can likewise suit a without dairy or veggie lover diet. Moreover, they all contain…

• NO gluten

• NO Sugar

• NO prepared grains

• NO soy

The remainder of the fixings are likewise healthy and regular and can be found in most typical supermarkets and on the web.

Moreover, they are all Paleo-accommodating, and each serving just contains 10 grams of net carbs or less, so these desserts are exceptionally adaptable and fit splendidly with a huge scope of diets. You can simply eat them in the event that you need healthier, and still similarly as flavorful, desserts that are quick and simple to make, and will assist you with getting more fit and control desires.

You've presumably known about the astounding weight reduction benefits of a ketogenic diet or "keto" for short. Since a keto diet contains almost no starch, it powers your body to utilize fat for energy, and overweight individuals normally lose a lot of muscle to fat ratio on the keto diet, without appetite or resolve.

Be that as it may, one issue with the keto diet can be removing sugar. You truly can't eat sugar on a keto diet. Hence, Kelsey made and accumulated recipes for 80 wanton desserts that adversary even the firsts, yet contain almost no sugar. How? Rather than the sugar, they contain some common and without calorie sugars that are made to taste precisely like genuine sugar, yet with fundamentally lower calories and effect on glucose and insulin levels. Accordingly, you can eat these desserts even on a keto diet and still be in ketosis, which is where you truly get the weight reduction benefits of the ketogenic diet.

So, what sorts of desserts will you have the option to prepare? What about…

- Almond spread brownie chomps.

- White chocolate raspberry cheesecake

- Classic vanilla Creme Brulee

- Chocolate secured bacon chomps (must attempt!)

- 7 sorts of dessert including chocolate almond frozen yogurt

- 8 sorts of cake including carrot cake

- 10 distinct cheesecakes

- 14 distinct confections

- 8 flaky, firm treat pies

- Much, considerably more!

What's extremely incredible is that practically all desserts were explicitly included to be quick and simple to make, and most can be made in under 15 minutes. There are, obviously, some increasingly included ones on the off chance that you truly need to dazzle your supper visitors, a date, or persuade somebody to give a shot the keto diet.

I can't over underscore how tasty these treats truly are. The cakes are soggy and fleecy, while the cakes are firm and chewy and delightful, much the same as they ought to be. Stunning.

It's likewise extremely simple to analyze a piece and make your own adaptations on the off chance that you feel like it, yet with 80 accomplished for-you recipes, you don't generally need to.

Another pleasant expansion is that, aside from the physical duplicate of the cookbook delivered to your entryway, you likewise get an advanced duplicate that you can download and utilize promptly and a few computerized rewards that will assist you with getting thinner and remain healthy with the keto diet.

In some cases, you need a keto to treat QUICK LIKE, and you would prefer not to need to cook anything or experience a major rigamarole to get you there. At the point when those minutes strike, you'll need to look through this rundown of the best keto no prepare desserts and discover something that will fulfill your keto sweet tooth STAT.

It's particularly essential to not need to cook or prepare your keto desserts throughout the mid-year months when it's blasting hot, and the exact opposite thing you need to do is turn the broiler or stove on.

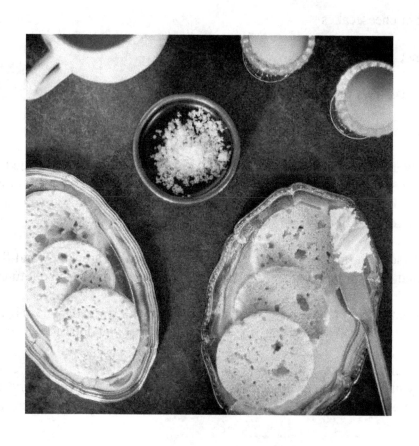

KETO DESSERTS RECIPES.

1. LOW CARB PECAN TURTLE TRUFFLES

These no-cook truffles are excessively simple to make so you can go from wanting to fulfill in not more than minutes! Sugar-free, low carb, keto cordial.

- Yield: 15 truffles

-

Category: Dessert

-

fixings

-

1/2 cup spread, softened

-

1/3 cup granulated sugar substitute (I utilized Swerve)

-

1/2 tsp caramel concentrate

-

1/4 tsp vanilla concentrate

-

1/3 cup zero carb vanilla protein powder

-

1 cup finely ground walnuts

-

4 squares Lindt 85% chocolate

-

15 walnut parts

directions

1.
Combine the spread, sugar, caramel, and vanilla concentrates, protein powder, and finely ground walnuts in a medium measured bowl. Blend well until completely joined.

2.
Roll into 15 truffles and spot them on wax or material paper.

3.
Melt the chocolate in a Ziploc sack in the microwave – around 1 moment. Cut the tip-off of one corner and press the chocolate onto the truffles.

4.
Press 1 walnut half into the highest point of every truffle.

5.   Chill. Serve.

notes

To see a rundown of my preferred low carb items and brands that I prescribe for sugars, flours, and so forth, you can look at the IBIH Pantry Ingredients Page!

nutrition

- Serving Size: per truffle

- Calories: 142

- Fat: 14

- Carbohydrates: 1g net

- Protein: 4

Espresso Panna Cotta with Raspberry Coulis – Low Carb and Gluten-Free

Smooth, rich espresso panna cotta made with Greek yogurt and showered with raspberry coulis. Low carb and sans gluten.

Fixings

Espresso Panna Cotta:

- 1 1/2 cups overwhelming cream isolated

- 1 envelope unflavoured gelatin

- 1 tbsp moment espresso

- 1/3 cup Swerve Sweetener

- 1 1/2 cups Greek yogurt I utilized full fat, yet you could do 2%

- 1/2 tsp vanilla concentrate

- 10 drops stevia extricate

Raspberry Coulis:

- 2 cups raspberries crisp or solidified (whenever solidified, defrost first)

- 3 tbsp powdered Swerve Sweetener

- 2 tsp crisp lemon juice

Guidelines

1.
For the panna cotta, gently oil 8 half-cup ramekins or serving dishes.

2.

Place 1/2 cup substantial cream into a medium pan, sprinkle gelatin over and let sit for 3 minutes.

3.
Add outstanding cream, moment espresso, and granulated erythritol, and set over medium warmth, racing until gelatin, espresso, and erythritol are disintegrated. Cook until blend starts to steam yet doesn't bubble.

4.
Remove from warmth and mix in Greek yogurt, vanilla and stevia until smooth.

5.
Divide between arranged ramekins, envelop by saran wrap, and chill in any event 3 hours.

6.
For the raspberry coulis, process raspberries and powdered erythritol in a food processor until pureed.

7.
Set a fine-work sifter over a bowl and channel, going ahead solids to get however much fluid through the strainer as could reasonably be expected. Mix in lemon juice.

8.
If you need to unmold your panna cotta, sit the ramekin in a few creeps of high temp water. At that point, run a sharp blade around the outside and upset onto a plate. Then again, you can leave it in the serving dish. Sprinkle with raspberry coulis and serve.

Formula Notes

Serves 8. Each serving has 6.5 g of carbs and 2 g of fiber. Complete NET CARBS = 4.5 g.

3. CHOCOLATE PEANUT BUTTER NO-BAKE COOKIES

-

Prep Time: 10 minutes

-

Total Time: 10 minutes

-

Yield: 10 Cookies 1x

Fixings

-

¼ cup rich, thick characteristic peanut spread

-

¼ cup rich, thick characteristic almond spread

-

3 tablespoons cream cheddar, mellowed

-

2 tablespoons salted margarine, dissolved

-

1 teaspoon unadulterated vanilla concentrate

-

2 tablespoons unsweetened cocoa powder

-

2 tablespoons confectioners erythritol, more to taste

- ¾ cup unsweetened dried up coconut

Guidelines

1.
Line a heating sheet with a silicone preparing mat or material paper.

2.
In a blending bowl, join the peanut spread, almond margarine, and cream cheddar. Blend until smooth.

3.

Add the margarine, vanilla concentrate, cocoa powder. Also, erythritol. Blend until all fixings are all around joined.

4.
Using an elastic spatula, crease in the coconut. Blend until it is equally circulated all through the blend.

5.   Drop 1/2 to 2-inch spoonfuls (10 aggregate) onto the readied preparing sheet.

6.
Freeze for 10 minutes before serving.

7.
Store additional items in the cooler until prepared to eat.

NOTES

Net carbs: 1.9g

NUTRITION

- Serving Size: 1 Cookie

- Calories: 132

- Sugar: 1.1g

- Sodium: 57mg

- Fat: 10.8g

- Carbohydrates: 4.4g

- Fiber: 2.5g

- Protein: 4.1g

4. LOW CARB KETO PUMPKIN COOKIES RECIPE

This chewy, delicate keto pumpkin cookies formula makes the ideal fall dessert! Perceive how to make healthy low carb pumpkin cookies with straightforward fixings and under 30 minutes.

Course Dessert

Calories 110 kcal

Planning Time 15 minutes

Cook Time 15 minutes

Complete Time 30 minutes

Servings cookies

Fixings

Pumpkin Cookies:

1/4 cup butter (unsalted)

1/3 cup Best Powdered Monk Fruit Erythritol Blend

1/2 cup pumpkin puree

1 huge Egg

1 tsp Vanilla concentrate

3 cups Blanched almond flour

2 tsp Cinnamon

1/2 tsp Nutmeg

1/2 tsp sans gluten preparing powder

1/4 tsp Sea salt

Discretionary Glaze/Frosting:

1/4 cup of besti Powdered Monk Fruit Erythritol Blend

1/4 cup of Heavy cream

1/4 tsp of Vanilla concentrate

Guidelines

1.   Preheat the broiler to 350 degrees F (176 degrees C). Line a huge preparing sheet with material paper.

2.   In an enormous profound bowl, beat together the spread and sugar until soft.

3.   Beat the pumpkin puree, the egg, and vanilla.

4.   Beat in the almond flour, cinnamon, nutmeg, heating powder, and ocean salt, until a uniform cookie batter structures.

5.   Use a medium cookie scoop to scoop chunks of mixture and pack the batter into it. Discharge onto the lined preparing sheet, 2 inches (5.08 cm) separated. Utilize your palm, or the base of a glass with a bending movement, to smooth cookies to around 1/4 inch (.64 cm) thick.

6.   Bake for 15 to 20 minutes, until brilliant.

7.   Meanwhile, make the coating/icing, if utilizing. In a little bowl, whisk together the coating fixings, until smooth. If that it's excessively thick, include more cream, a teaspoon at once, until it's a spreadable consistency.

8.   When it is done, spread a teaspoon of coating on every cookie (or basically sprinkle with powdered sugar). Cool totally to solidify before moving from the container.

Formula NOTES

Serving size: 1 2-inch cookie

NUTRITION INFORMATION PER SERVING

Nutrition Facts

Sum per serving. Serving size in formula notes above.

Calories110

Fat9g

Protein3g

Absolute Carbs4g

Net Carbs3g

Fiber1g

Sugar0g

5. LOW CARB PALEO KETO CHOCOLATE MUG CAKE RECIPE

Perceive how to make a keto mug cake in a short time, utilizing 6 fixings! This rich, clammy, low carb paleo chocolate mug cake formula has just 4 grams net carbs.

Course Dessert

.

Calories 433 kcal

Planning Time 2 minutes

Cook Time 2 minutes

All out Time 4 minutes

Servings mug cake

Fixings

1 tbsp Butter (salted; *see notes for sans dairy choices)

3/4 oz Unsweetened heating chocolate

3 tbsp Blanched almond flour

1 1/2 tbsp Besti Monk Fruit Allulose Blend (or any granulated sugar; *see notes for choices)

1/2 tsp sans gluten preparing powder

1 enormous Egg

1/4 tsp Vanilla concentrate (discretionary)

Guidelines

Microwave Instructions

1. Disolve the margarine and chocolate together in a mug or huge 12 oz (355 mL) ramekin in the microwave (around 45-60 seconds, blending part of the way through). Be mindful so as not to consume it. Ensure the ramekin is at any rate twofold the volume of the fixings, in light of the fact that the mug cake will rise.

2.
Add the almond flour, sugar, heating powder, egg, and vanilla (if utilizing). Mix everything great until totally combined.

3.
Microwave for around 60-75 seconds, until simply firm. (Try not to overcook, or it will be dry.)

4. Serve it with the whipped cream, or potentially shower with increasingly dissolved chocolate mixed with sugar.

Broiler Instructions

1.
Preheat the broiler to 350 degrees F (177 degrees C).

2.
Melt the margarine and chocolate together in a twofold heater on the stove. Be mindful so as not to consume it. Expel from heat.

3.
Add the almond flour, sugar, heating powder, egg, and vanilla (if utilizing). Mix everything great until totally combined.

4.
Transfer the player to an enormous 12 oz (355 mL) stove safe ramekin (or two littler 6 oz (178 mL) ones). Ensure the ramekins are at any rate twofold the volume of the fixings, on the grounds that the cake will rise. Heat for around 15 minutes, until simply firm.

5.
Serve with whipped cream (or coconut whipped cream for paleo), as well as sprinkle with increasingly dissolved chocolate mixed with sugar.

Formula NOTES

Serving size: 1 mug cake (whole formula)

•

For a sans dairy or paleo rendition, use ghee or coconut oil, and include a spot of salt.

•

The unique variant of this formula utilized erythritol; however, the priest organic product allulose mix makes a far unrivaled, very damp mug cake. Paleo devotees may want to utilize coconut sugar for the sugar.

NUTRITION INFORMATION PER SERVING

Nutrition Facts

Sum per serving. Serving size in formula notes above.

Calories433

Fat38g

Protein14g

Absolute Carbs11g

Net Carbs4g

Fiber7g

Sugar1g

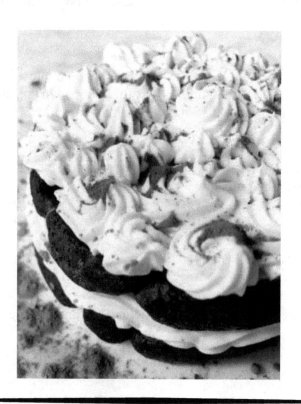

6. LOW CARB KETO APPLE PIE RECIPE

This keto crusty fruit-filled treat formula possesses a flavor like the genuine article! With a mystery fixing keto crusty fruit-filled treat filling and an almond flour outside layer, a without sugar low carb crusty fruit-filled treat truly is conceivable.

Course Dessert

.

Calories 363 kcal

Planning Time 25 minutes

Cook Time 1 hour 10 minutes

Cooling Time 20 minutes

Absolute Time 1 hour 35 minutes

Servings

Fixings

Keto Apple Pie Filling:

    1/2 cup of butter (salted)

    1/4 cup of Besti Powdered Monk Fruit Erythritol Blend (or more to taste)

    6 tbsp of Lemon juice (partitioned)

    2 tsp of Cinnamon

    1 tsp of nutmeg

    1/2 tsp of Cardamom

    1 tbsp of gelatin-powder

    5 medium Yellow squash of (6-7 cups, ~50 oz, cut and diced into 1/2 inch pieces; or zucchini!)

1 tsp of Vanilla concentrate (discretionary)

1/2 tsp Maple remove (discretionary)

Keto Apple Pie Crust:

    3 3/4 cup of blanched almond flour

    1/3 cup of besti Monk Fruit Erythritol Blend

    1/2 tsp of Sea salt

    1/2 cup of Butter

    1 enormous Egg

    1/2 tsp Vanilla concentrate (discretionary)

1 tbsp Unflavored gelatin powder

2 tbsp Water

Guidelines

Keto Apple Pie Filling:

1.
In a little squeeze bowl, whisk the gelatin powder with 3 tablespoons (44 mL) lemon juice. Put aside to sprout.

2.
In a huge 3.5-quart (3.3 liters) pot, soften the margarine over medium warmth. Mix in the powdered sugar, the staying 3 tablespoons (44 mL) lemon juice, cinnamon, nutmeg, and cardamom. At the point when the gelatin blend has thickened, whisk it into the container, until broken up.

3.
Add the diced squash to the dish. Bring to a stew. Stew over medium warmth for around 30-40 minutes, until the squash is extremely delicate and the blend has thickened, like crusty fruit-filled treat filling.

4.
Stir in the maple separate.

5.   Set the filling to cool until no more sultry than tepid, at any rate, 20 minutes.

Keto Apple Pie Crust:

1.   Meanwhile, preheat the broiler to 350 degrees F (177 degrees C).

2.   To make the pie outside layer mixture, follow stages 1-3 from this almond flour pie hull formula, BUT you will utilize the measures of almond flour, sugar, ocean salt, margarine, egg, and vanilla above.

3.   Add the gelatin powder and water, and utilize a hand blender to join, until uniform.

4.   Divide the batter into equal parts. Press half of the batter into the lined pie skillet, including the base and going up the sides. Set the second 50% of the batter aside.

5.   Bake the hull in the broiler for 10-12 minutes, until just daintily brilliant.

6.   When done, put aside to cool for in any event 10 minutes before including the filling.

7.   Meanwhile, place the staying half of the batter between two softly oiled bits of material paper. Utilize a turning pin over the material paper to turn out to a circle marginally bigger than the highest point of the pie container, for the top hull.

Keto Apple Pie Assembly:

1.   Preheat the broiler again to 350 degrees F (177 degrees C), in the event that it has cooled. Ensure the filling and base covering are both cooled to no more smoking than tepid before collecting.

2.
Gently exchange the cooled filling to the cooled base outside layer.

3.
Lift the top bit of material paper off the turned out top outside. Utilizing the base bit of material paper, cautiously and quickly flip the top covering over onto the pie, at that point delicately strip off the material paper. Utilize a blade to cut any abundance top outside off the edges, ensuring it still totally covers the base hull. Utilize your fingers to press the edges down to seal. Cut 4 cuts in the highest point of the pie.

4.Spread the edges of the pie with thwart and heat for an extra 5-15 minutes, until the top outside layer is light brilliant and semi-firm to the touch. (It won't completely firm up until subsequent to cooling.)

5.   Remove the pie from the stove and cool totally before cutting or expelling from the container.

Formula NOTES

Serving size: 1 cut, or 1/12 of the whole formula

NUTRITION INFORMATION PER SERVING

Nutrition Facts

Sum per serving. Serving size in formula notes above.

Calories363

Fat33g

Protein10g

Absolute Carbs12g

Net Carbs8g

Fiber4g

Sugar3g

7. BLACKBERRY SUGAR-FREE KETO FROZEN YOGURT RECIPE

Figure out how to make keto solidified yogurt - the ideal healthy treat. Simple solidified Greek yogurt takes only 5 minutes + 4 fixings!

Course Dessert

.

Calories 63 kcal

Planning Time 5 minutes

Freezing 2 hours

Complete Time 5 minutes

Servings

Fixings

4 cups Blackberries (solidified)

1 cup of Greek yogurt (full-fat)

1 tbsp Lemon juice

1 tsp Vanilla concentrate

Directions

1.   Put it into the blender and mix till smooth.

2.
Place in a cooler safe compartment and freeze for in any event 2 hours, or until your ideal consistency is come to.

Formula NOTES

Serving size: 1/6 of the formula (~3/4 cup)

NUTRITION INFORMATION PER SERVING

Nutrition Facts

Sum per serving. Serving size in formula notes above.

Calories63

Fat0g

Protein4g

All out Carbs10g

Net Carbs5g

Fiber5g

Sugar5g

8. Simple SUGAR-FREE POPSICLES RECIPE: BLUEBERRY LEMON POPSICLES

Figure out how to make sans sugar popsicles (blueberry lemon popsicles!) in only 5 minutes + 4 fixings! This simple without sugar popsicle formula is healthy and delightful.

Course Dessert

.

Calories 56 kcal

Planning Time 5 minutes

Complete Time 4 hours 5 minutes

Servings popsicles

Fixings

1 1/2 cup Blueberries

   1/3 cup of besti Powdered Monk Fruit

   1/4 cup Lemon juice

   1/4 cup Full-fat coconut cream

Directions

1.   Puree all fixings in a blender—taste and change sugar as wanted.

2.   Pour the blend into popsicle molds. Freeze for around 4 hours, until strong.

Formula NOTES

Serving size: 1 popsicle

NUTRITION INFORMATION PER SERVING

Nutrition Facts

Sum per serving. Serving size in formula notes above.

Calories56

Fat3g

Protein0g

Absolute Carbs7g

Net Carbs6g

Fiber1g

Sugar4g

9. THE SUGAR-FREE KETO & LOW CARB WITH CREAM CHEESE

Low carb key lime pie with cream cheddar (avocado key lime pie) is DELICIOUSLY rich and reviving! Only 10 minutes prep + 7 elements for this simple keto key lime pie formula.

Course Dessert

.

Calories 324 kcal

Planning Time 10 minutes

Chilling Time 2 hours

Absolute Time 10 minutes

Servings cuts

Fixings

Outside

- 2 cups Blanched almond flour

- 1/3 cup Coconut oil (liquefied)

- 2 tbsp Besti Monk Fruit Allulose Blend

- Filling

- 2 medium Avocado (ready)

- 12 oz Cream cheddar (mellowed at room temperature or by heating)

- 4 little Limes

- 2/3 cup of besti Powdered Monk Fruit Allulose Blend

- 1 tsp of Vanilla concentrate

Directions

1.
Line the base of a pie container with material paper (discretionary, however, makes it simpler to expel the cuts later).

2.
To make the outside layer, mix together the almond flour, coconut oil, and sugar. Press the outside layer into the pie skillet. Put in a safe spot.

3.   Place the avocado (skin expelled), relaxed cream cheddar, powdered sugar, and vanilla concentrate into a powerful blender or a food processor.

4.
Zest the limes utilizing a zester and add the get-up-and-go to the blender. Crush the juice out of the considerable number of limes in there also. Puree the blend until smooth, scratching down the sides with a spatula.

5.
Pour/spoon the pureed blend into the outside. Smooth with a spatula or the rear of a spoon.

6.
Refrigerate for in any event two hours, until the pie is firm. Present with natively constructed sans sugar whipped cream whenever wanted. Keep refrigerated.

Formula NOTES

Serving size: 1 cut, or 1/12 of the whole pie

NUTRITION INFORMATION PER SERVING

Nutrition Facts

Sum per serving. Serving size in formula notes above.

Calories324

Fat31g

Protein7g

All out Carbs9g

Net Carbs5g

Fiber4g

Sugar1g

10. LOW CARB-KETO ICE CREAM RECIPE (SUGAR-FREE)

Perceive how to make a keto dessert with only 4 fixings! It's the best without low sugar carb dessert formula I've at any point made. It is so natural to make this keto well-disposed dessert formula.

Course Dessert

.

Calories 347 kcal

Planning Time 5 minutes

Cook Time 30 minutes

All out Time 5 hours 35 minutes

Servings

Fixings

3 tbsp Butter

3 cups Heavy cream (isolated into 2c and 1c - see notes)

1/3 cup Powdered allulose

1 tsp Vanilla concentrate

1/4 cup of MCT Oil (or MCT oil powder; one of these is enthusiastically suggested if not utilizing a dessert creator)

1 medium Vanilla bean (discretionary; seeds scratched)

Directions

The most effective method to Make Low Carb Ice Cream (For BOTH Methods - No Churn or Ice Cream Maker)

1.   Melt the spread in an enormous pot over medium warmth. Include 2/3 of the overwhelming cream (2 cups (473 mL)) and powdered sugar. Heat to the point of boiling, at that point, decrease to a stew. Stew for 30-45 minutes, blending every so often, until the blend is thick, covers the rear of a spoon, and volume is diminished considerably. It will likewise pull away from the dish as you tilt it. (This will speed up on the off chance that you utilize a bigger skillet.)

2.   Pour into a huge bowl and permit to cool to room temperature. Mix in the vanilla concentrate, and seeds from the vanilla bean, if utilizing. Speed in the MCT oil or MCT oil powder if utilizing - this is energetically suggested all in all, and an unquestionable requirement in the event that you don't have a frozen yogurt creator.

3.   Whisk the staying 1 cup overwhelming cream into the sweet blend in the bowl, until smooth.

The most effective method to Make Keto Ice Cream With An Ice Cream Maker

1.   Transfer the blend to your frozen yogurt producer and stir as indicated by maker's guidelines, until the dessert is the consistency of delicate serve. (My frozen yogurt creator took 15-20 minutes.)

2.   Enjoy promptly, or move to a cooler holder and freeze for 2-4 hours, until firm.

The most effective method to Make Keto Ice Cream Without An Ice Cream Maker

1.
Transfer the blend to a cooler compartment (like a 9x5 in (23x13 cm) portion container) and smooth the top with a spatula. (If you need to include blend ins, delicately mix them in at this progression, and furthermore sprinkle some on top.) Line the surface with a bit of material or wax paper to keep ice gems from shaping. (You can utilize a frozen yogurt creator in the event that you have one.)

2.
Freeze for 5-6 hours, until firm. Mix the frozen yogurt during the freezing procedure, at regular intervals for the initial 2 hours and each 60-an hour and a half for 2-3 hours after. (Dessert will get hard in the cooler after longer time frames. Let it relax on the counter for 10-30 minutes before serving, and utilize a wet dessert scoop to serve.)

Formula NOTES

Serving size: 1/2 cup

- This keto frozen yogurt formula was refreshed in June 2018 and again in July 2019 to improve the surface. The progressions included fixing sums and technique. However, nutrition information has not changed a lot. Nutrition information underneath mirrors the present without sugar frozen yogurt formula appeared here, excluding discretionary MCT oil/powder. The still shows the old technique for whipping the cream, which you don't have to do - simply whisk the fluid legitimately into the consolidated milk.

- If you'd prefer to help up the without sugar dessert a piece, you can supplant a portion of the overwhelming cream in stage 1 with coconut milk or almond milk rather (it might take more time to lessen). Be that as it may, you would prefer not to supplant any of the creams in stage 4.

- Low carb dessert hardens if it's in the cooler excessively long. Utilizing MCT oil or MCT oil powder in the formula makes a difference.

- After more than 6-8 hours in the cooler, you will probably need to relax without sugar frozen yogurt on the counter before serving.

NUTRITION INFORMATION PER SERVING

Nutrition Facts

Sum per serving. Serving size in formula notes above.

Calories347

Fat36g

Protein2g

Complete Carbs3g

Net Carbs3g

Fiber0g

Sugar2g

11. FROZEN KETO-LOW CARB PEANUT BUTTER PIE RECIPE

Perceive how to make the most wanton keto low carb peanut margarine pie! This simple solidified no prepare peanut spread pie formula has 5g net carbs + needs only 15 minutes prep.

Course Dessert

.

Calories 304 kcal

Planning Time 15 minutes

Chilling Time 1 hour 35 minutes

All out Time 15 minutes

Servings

Fixings

Outside layer:

2 bundles Nui peanut margarine cookies (4 cookies)

1 bundle Nui twofold chocolate cookies (2 cookies)

1/4 cup Butter (salted, cool, cut into little pieces)

2 tbsp Powdered allulose

Filling:

3/4 cup Peanut margarine (smooth characteristic)

4 oz Cream cheddar (relaxed)

1/3 cup Powdered allulose

1 tsp Vanilla concentrate

1 1/8 cup Heavy cream (isolated into 6 tbsp and 3/4 cup)

Guidelines

1.
Place the cookies into a food processor. Heartbeat until they are the consistency of morsels.

2.
Add the margarine and powdered sugar and heartbeat once more, just until uniform and brittle.

3.
Chill the mixture in the ice chest for around 15 minutes, until it's less clingy and sufficiently simple to work with.

4.   Press the cookie mixture dish and up the sides of a 9-inch (23 cm) pie skillet, to frame the outside layer.

5.
Freeze the outside layer for 20 minutes.

6.
Meanwhile, in an enormous, profound bowl, beat together the peanut spread, cream cheddar, and powdered sugar for around 2 minutes, until fleecy. Beat in the vanilla concentrate. Beat in roughly 6 tablespoons (88 mL) substantial cream, 1 tablespoon (15 mL) at once, until it arrives at the consistency of thick icing. The measure of cream you need will fluctuate contingent upon how thick your peanut spread was, so simply continue including 1 tablespoon (15 mL) at once until it resembles a thick icing.

7.
In a subsequent bowl, beat 3/4 cup (177 mL) overwhelming cream until firm pinnacles structure. Crease the whipped cream into the peanut margarine blend.

8.
Transfer the filling into the pie container over the outside layer.

9.
Freeze for in any event 60 minutes, until firm. Keep solidified, yet let it sit on the counter to mellow somewhat if it's excessively hard right out of the cooler (like a frozen yogurt cake). On the off chance that you like garnishes, you can include liquefied peanut margarine shower, dissolved chocolate sprinkle, or potentially more Nui cookies disintegrated on top (these are discretionary).

Formula NOTES

Serving size: 1 cut, 1/12 of the whole formula

NUTRITION INFORMATION PER SERVING

Nutrition Facts

Sum per serving. Serving size in formula notes above.

Calories304

Fat28g

Protein6g

Absolute Carbs7g

Net Carbs5g

Fiber2g

Sugar2g

12. KETO LOW CARB MILKSHAKE RECIPE - VANILLA

This keto milkshake formula (sans sugar milkshake) is EASY and only 4 fixings!

Course Dessert

Calories 379 kcal

Planning Time 5 minutes

All out Time 5 minutes

Servings

Fixings

1 13.5-oz would coconut be able to drain (cold; utilize just cream and dispose of coconut water)

1 cup of heavy cream (or more coconut milk/cream for sans dairy/paleo)

1/4 cup of besti Powdered Monk Fruit Allulose Blend

2 tsp Vanilla concentrate

2 cups Ice shapes

Guidelines

1.
In a blender, mix together everything aside from ice for 20 seconds.

2.
Add ice shapes. Heartbeat again until the ice is simply squashed, however not longer (it might get watery on the off chance that you mix excessively).

Formula NOTES

Serving size: 1 cup

NUTRITION INFORMATION PER SERVING

Nutrition Facts

Sum per serving. Serving size in formula notes above.

Calories379

Fat38g

Protein3g

Absolute Carbs4g

Net Carbs4g

Fiber0g

Sugar3g

13. KETO LOW CARB RICOTTA DESSERT RECIPE

Figure out how to make low carb ricotta dessert (keto berry dessert) in only 10 minutes. This simple keto ricotta sweet will get one of your new most loved ricotta cheddar dessert recipes - no sugar required!

Course Dessert

Cooking Italian

Calories 202 kcal

Planning Time 10 minutes

Servings

Fixings

1 1/2 lb Whole milk ricotta

1/4 cup Heavy cream

1 tbsp Lemon get-up-and-go (or 2 tbsp for more lemon-y season)

1/2 cup Powdered erythritol

2 tsp Vanilla concentrate

1 cup Raspberries

1 cup Blueberries

1 cup Blackberries

Directions

1.
In a blender, consolidate the ricotta, overwhelming cream, lemon get-up-and-go, powdered sugar, and vanilla. Puree until smooth.

2.
In 4 parfait cups, manufacture rotating layers of ricotta whip and 1/4 cup (32 grams) of each sort of berries.

3.
If wanted, embellish with whipped cream and additional berries.

Formula NOTES

Serving size: 1/2 parfait cup

Note: I utilized enormous parfait cups, so 1/2 is bounty filling for a pastry serving. You can utilize little ones (or fill bigger ones midway) in the event that you need it to be progressively helpful to have a whole cup be a serving.

NUTRITION INFORMATION PER SERVING

Nutrition Facts

Sum per serving. Serving size in formula notes above.

Calories202

Fat13g

Protein10g

All out Carbs9g

Net Carbs7g

Fiber2g

Sugar4g

14. THE BEST KETO SUGAR-FREE CHOCOLATE PUDDING RECIPE

A rich, without sugar low carb chocolate pudding formula that preferences superior to locally acquired! Perceive how to make keto chocolate pudding with 5 fixings + 10 minutes prep.

Course Dessert

.

Calories 431 kcal

Planning Time 5 minutes

Cook Time 5 minutes

Chill Time 2 hours

All out Time 10 minutes

Servings

Fixings

2 cups Heavy cream (partitioned into 1/4 cup and 1 3/4 cup)

1 1/2 tsp Unflavored gelatin powder

1/3 cup Powdered erythritol

1/4 cup Cocoa powder

1/4 tsp Sea salt

2 tsp Vanilla concentrate

Directions

1.
Pour 1/4 cup overwhelming cream into a little bowl. Sprinkle the gelatin powder on top (don't simply dump it in), and whisk together right away. Put in a safe spot.

2.
In a medium pot over medium-low, mix together the staying overwhelming cream, powdered sugar, cocoa powder, and ocean salt. Warmth, whisking continually, for about5 minutes, until the blend is smooth and rising close to the edges.

3.
Remove from heat. Mix in the vanilla concentrate.

4.   Add the gelatin to the skillet. Race until smooth and broke down.

5.
Let the pudding cool for around 10 minutes, until cooled enough not to soften plastic wrap to be set over it. Whisk again to dispose of any film on top.

6.
Cover with saran wrap flush against the top to keep a film from shaping. Refrigerate for in any event 2 hours, until firm.

Formula NOTES

Serving size: 1/2 cup

Note: This keto pudding is VERY rich! Cut the serving size down the middle for a lighter treat that is still very fulfilling.

!

NUTRITION INFORMATION PER SERVING

Nutrition Facts

Sum per serving. Serving size in formula notes above.

Calories431

Fat43g

Protein5g

Absolute Carbs6g

Net Carbs5g

Fiber1g

Sugar3g

15. Simple LOW CARB KETO CUSTARD RECIPE

A 5-fixing vanilla keto custard formula! Keto egg custard is excessively EASY. Furthermore, this low carb custard formula is an ideal sweet for making ahead.

Course Dessert

Cooking French

Calories 303 kcal

Planning Time 5 minutes

Cook Time 35 minutes

Absolute Time 40 minutes

Servings

Fixings

2 huge Eggs

2 cups Heavy cream

1/2 cup Powdered erythritol (1/2 cup Powdered erythritol)

1/4 tsp Sea salt

2 tsp Vanilla concentrate

Nutmeg (discretionary, for sprinkling)

Directions

1.   Pre-heat the cooker to 350 degrees F (177 degrees C).

2.   In a medium bowl, beat the eggs at medium-low speed for around 30 seconds until foamy.

3.
In a little pot, join the cream, powdered erythritol, and ocean salt over medium-low warmth. Warmth, mixing incidentally, for a couple of moments until it arrives at 180 degrees F (82 degrees C), or not long before bubbling. Little air pockets will frame on the edges. Try not to allow it to bubble. Mix in the vanilla concentrate.

4.
While whisking the eggs continually, empty the cream into the eggs gradually in a slight stream.

5.
Divide the custard blend uniformly between 6 4-ounce ramekins. Sprinkle the tops softly with nutmeg.

6.

Place the ramekins into a container with tall sides, and fill the skillet with enough water to arrive at most of the way up the sides of the ramekins.

7.
Bake for 30 to 40 minutes, until the custard, is scarcely beginning to set, yet jiggly. A blade embedded in the inside should tell the truth.

8.
Cool the custard totally to room temperature until set. Refrigerate subsequently if serving later.

Formula NOTES

Serving size: 1 4-ounce ramekin

NUTRITION INFORMATION PER SERVING

Nutrition Facts

Sum per serving. Serving size in formula notes above.

Calories303

Fat30g

Protein4g

Absolute Carbs2g

Net Carbs2g

Fiber0g

Sugar2g

16. CRUSTLESS LOW CARB KETO CHEESECAKE BITES RECIPE (CHEESECAKE FAT BOMBS)

Keto cheesecake chomps + cheesecake fat bombs in one - only 1 NET CARB each! You just need 6 fixings required for this smaller than normal low carb cheesecake nibbles formula.

Course Dessert

.

Calories 72 kcal

Planning Time 10 minutes

Cook Time 15 minutes

Chilling Time 60 minutes

Absolute Time 25 minutes

Servings

Fixings

Cheesecake chomps:

16 oz Cream cheddar (mellowed)

1 huge Egg (at room temperature)

1 tsp Lemon juice

1/2 tsp Vanilla concentrate

1/2 cup Besti Powdered Monk Fruit Allulose Blend

Raspberry twirl:

4 oz Raspberries

1 1/2 tbsp Water

4 tsp Besti Powdered Monk Fruit Allulose Blend

Discretionary fixings:

Whipped cream (unsweetened or with without sugar)

24 Raspberries

Directions

1.   Preheat the cooker to 350 degrees F (177 degrees C). Line a smaller than normal biscuit skillet with 24 material liners.

2.
Place the raspberries, water, and powdered sugar into an exceptionally little pot. Warmth over low warmth until the raspberries begin to relax, around 2 to 3 minutes.

3.   Stew for a couple of more minutes, until the sauce thickens.

4.
Using a hand blender or stand blender, beat the cream cheddar and powdered sugar together at low to medium speed until fleecy.

5.
Beat in the egg; at that point, the lemon juice and vanilla concentrate. (Keep the blender at low to medium the entire time; too fast will present too many air bubbles, which we don't need.)

6.
Spoon the cheesecake filling equitably into the biscuit liners.

7.
Spoon a 1/2 teaspoon (2.5 mL) of raspberry sauce over each cream cheddar cup. Utilize a toothpick to whirl into the hitter.

8.   Bake it for 10-15 minutes, until the chomps are puffed up and nearly set, yet at the same time jiggly.

9.
Remove the cheesecake chomps from the broiler. They may fall, which is typical. Cool totally at room temperature, at that point chill for at any rate 60 minutes, until firm and cold.

10.
To serve, pipe a spot of sans sugar whipped cream into the focal point of each chomp and top with a crisp raspberry.

Formula NOTES

Serving size: 1 cheesecake nibble

NUTRITION INFORMATION PER SERVING

Nutrition Facts

Sum per serving. Serving size in formula notes above.

Calories72

Fat6g

Protein1g

All out Carbs1g

Net Carbs1g

Fiber0g

Sugar0g

17. KETO LOW CARB LEMON BARS RECIPE

This low carb lemon bars formula is ideal for spring, and I'm sharing my tips for PERFECT keto lemon bars unfailingly. These without sugar lemon bars have only 7 fixings!

Course Dessert

.

Calories 166 kcal

Planning Time 10 minutes

Cook Time 28 minutes

Chilling Time 2 hours

Absolute Time 38 minutes

Servings

Fixings

Shortbread outside:

    2 1/2 cups of lanched almond flour

    1/4 cup of besti Monk Fruit Allulose Blend

1/4 tsp of Sea salt

1/4 cup of coconut oil (liquefied)

1 huge Egg (whisked)

1/2 tsp Vanilla concentrate

Lemon filling:

1/3 cup of besti Powdered Monk Fruit Allulose Blend

1/4 cup of blanched almond flour

4 huge Eggs

3/4 cup of Lemon juice

1 tbsp of lemon get-up-and-go

Directions

1.   Preheat the cooker to 350 degrees F (177 degrees C). Line 9x9 inch (23x23 cm) container with material paper hanging over the sides.

2.   Make the filling first, since it must be all set quickly when the outside leaves the broiler. I
3.   Mix the eggs, lemon juice, and lemon pizzazz, until smooth. Put in a safe spot.

4.
To make the covering, join the almond flour, sugar, and ocean salt in an enormous bowl.

5.
Stir in the dissolved coconut oil, at that point, the egg and vanilla. The batter will be brittle, yet ready to be squeezed together.

6.
Press the batter into the lined container. Prepare for around 13 to 16 minutes, until firm and brilliant.

7.
Remove the hull from the stove, and promptly pour the filling over the outside layer.

8.
Return to the stove for 15 to 18 minutes, until filling is set, yet at the same time delicate.

9.

Cool totally on the counter, without moving or cutting. Cover and refrigerate for in any event 2 hours before cutting.

Formula

Serving : 1/16 of the whole formula

NUTRITION INFORMATION PER SERVING

Nutrition Facts

Sum per serving. Serving size in formula notes above.

Calories166

Fat14g

Protein6g

Absolute Carbs5g

Net Carbs3g

Fiber2g

Sugar1g

18. LOW CARB KETO TIRAMISU RECIPE

A definitive low carb tiramisu formula - the ideal harmony among real and simple! This keto tiramisu pastry is a wanton make-ahead treat.

Course Dessert

Cooking Italian

Calories 408 kcal

Planning Time 20 minutes

Cook Time 40 minutes

Absolute Time 60 minutes

Servings

Fixings

Cake:

  1/3 cup of Besti Monk Fruit Erythritol Blend

  1/3 cup of Butter (mellowed)

  3 big eggs (at room temperature)

  1/4 cup of heavy cream (at room temperature)

  1 tsp Vanilla concentrate

1 1/2 cups Blanched almond flour

1 tsp without gluten preparing powder

1/8 tsp Sea salt

Shower:

1/4 mug Espresso (or solid espresso, at room temperature)

2 tbsp Brandy (or cognac, discretionary)

Filling:

4 huge Egg yolks (at room temperature)

3 tbsp Besti Powdered Monk Fruit Erythritol Blend

1 cup Mascarpone (at room temperature)

1 cup Heavy cream (cold)

1/2 tsp Cocoa powder (discretionary, for cleaning)

Directions

Cake:

1.   Preheat the cooker to 350 degrees F (177 degrees C). Line a 9 in (23 cm) square container with material paper, so it hangs over the sides.

2.   Beat the sugar and margarine until fleecy.

3.
Beat in the eggs; at that point, the overwhelming cream and vanilla concentrate.

4.
Beat in the almond flour, preparing powder, and salt, until smooth.

5.
Transfer the batter to the fixed container and smooth the top with a spatula.

6.   Bake for 20-25 min., until firm, brilliant, and an embedded toothpick tells the truth.

Filling:

1.
Meanwhile, make the filling. Consolidate the egg yolks and powdered sugar in the highest point of a little twofold kettle, over bubbling water. (Ensure the twofold heater bowl is little.) Reduce warmth to low, and cook for around 7 to 10 minutes, mixing continually, until the blend is lighter in shading, expanded in volume, and somewhat foamy.

2.
Remove from heat. Utilize a hand blender at medium-low speed to whip the yolks until they are thick and lemon in shading. Put aside to cool while doing the subsequent stage.

3.
In a different bowl, whip the substantial cream at rapid until firm pinnacles structure.

4.
Add the mascarpone to the whipped yolks. Beat at low speed until joined easily.

5.
Gently overlay the mascarpone yolk blend into the whipped cream.

Gathering:

1.
Run a blade along the edges of the cake to ensure it didn't adhere to the sides. Move to a cutting board.

2. In a little small bowl, mix together the coffee and cognac. Pour uniformly over the cake.

3.
Cut the cake down the middle, framing 2 square shapes. Cautiously slide one half onto a platter.

4. Cautiously place the second 50% of the cake on top, at that point top with the rest of the cream blend.

5.
Sift cocoa powder through a fine-work sifter over the tiramisu (discretionary).

6.
Refrigerate for 4 hours, or ideally medium-term, to set.

Formula NOTES

Serving size: 1/10 of the whole cake, either a cut just about an inch thick or a square around 1.8 x 2.25 inches.

NUTRITION INFORMATION PER SERVING

Nutrition Facts

Sum per serving. Serving size in formula notes above.

Calories408

Fat38g

Protein9g

All out Carbs6g

Net Carbs5g

Fiber1g

Sugar1g

19. RASPBERRY LOW CARB KETO CHIA PUDDING RECIPE WITH ALMOND MILK

Simple keto chia pudding quickly - only 6 fixings! Medium-term raspberry chia pudding with almond milk is such a great amount of superior to plain low carb chia pudding.

Course Breakfast

.

Calories 337 kcal

Planning Time 5 minutes

Chill 12 hours

Absolute Time 5 minutes

Servings serving

Fixings

1/2 cup Raspberries

1/4 cup Chia seeds

2 tbsp Vital Proteins Collagen Peptides

1 tbsp Powdered erythritol

3/4 cup unsweetened almond milk

1/4 tsp Vanilla concentrate

Directions

1.
Mash the raspberries in a little bowl.

2.

In another bowl, mix together the chia seeds, collagen, and powdered sugar.

3.

Stir in the almond milk, at that point the vanilla and squashed raspberries.

4.

Chill medium-term. Mix again before serving.

Formula NOTES

Serving size: Entire formula, around 1/2 cup

NUTRITION INFORMATION PER SERVING

Nutrition Facts

Sum per serving. Serving size in formula notes above.

Calories337

Fat15g

Protein26g

All out Carbs25g

Net Carbs6g

Fiber19g

Sugar2g

KETO LOW CARB NO-BAKE CHOCOLATE CHEESECAKE RECIPE

A simple no heat chocolate cheesecake formula with brief prep! Keto low carb chocolate cheesecake has only 5 fixings in the outside layer and 4 in the filling.

Course Dessert

.

Calories 238 kcal

Planning Time 20 minutes

Refrigerate 2 hours

All out Time 2 hours 20 minutes

Servings

Fixings

- Low Carb Chocolate Cheesecake Crust:

- 1 3/4 cup Blanched almond flour

- 3 tbsp Cocoa powder

- 3 tbsp Besti Monk Fruit Erythritol Blend

- 1/3 cup Butter (liquefied)

- 1 tsp Vanilla concentrate

Low Carb Chocolate Cheesecake Filling:

- 8 oz Unsweetened heating chocolate

- 24 oz Cream cheddar

- 1 1/4 cup of Besti Powdered Monk Fruit Erythritol Blend

- 1 tsp of Vanilla concentrate

Guidelines

Low Carb Chocolate Cheesecake Crust:

1.   In an enormous bowl, mix together the almond flour, cocoa powder, and erythritol.

2.   In a little bowl, mix together the liquefied margarine and vanilla. Add to the almond flour blend. Mix well, squeezing with the rear of a spoon or spatula until uniform. It ought to be brittle, yet clingy enough to press together.

3.   Press the no-heat outside layer into the base of the dish. Chill while setting up the filling.

Low Carb Chocolate Cheesecake Filling:

1.   Dissolve the unsweetened chocolate in the microwave or a twofold kettle on the stove, blending sporadically. Be mindful so as not to overheat. Put aside to cool.

2.   Meanwhile, utilize a hand blender at medium-low speed to beat together the cream cheddar, powdered sugar, and vanilla concentrate, until cushioned and uniform. Beat in the vanilla.

3.   When the chocolate has cooled to warm, however no longer hot, beat into the cream at medium-low speed.

4.
Transfer the filling to the outside layer and utilize a spatula to cover it up. Refrigerate for at any rate 2 hours, until set.

Formula NOTES

Serving size: 1 cut, or 1/12 of the whole cheesecake

NUTRITION INFORMATION PER SERVING

Nutrition Facts

Sum per serving. Serving size in formula notes above.

Calories238

Fat23g

Protein6g

Complete Carbs10g

Net Carbs5g

Fiber5g

Sugar0g

20. GLUTEN-FREE KETO COCONUT MACAROONS RECIPE

The best without gluten keto coconut macaroons formula takes only 25 minutes! Figure out how to make coconut macaroons with only 6 fixings + one bowl.

Course Dessert

Cooking Italian

Calories 135 kcal

Planning Time 10 minutes

Cook Time 15 minutes

Chilling Time 20 minutes

Absolute Time 25 minutes

Servings macaroons

Fixings

2 huge Egg whites (at room temperature)

1/3 cup Besti Monk Fruit Allulose Blend

1 tsp Vanilla concentrate (or a mix of vanilla and almond removes)

1/4 tsp Sea salt

2 cups Unsweetened destroyed coconut

2 oz without sugar Dark Chocolate Chips (discretionary)

1/2 tbsp Coconut oil (discretionary)

Guidelines

1.   Preheat the broiler to 325 degrees F (163 degrees C). Line a preparing sheet with material paper.

2.   Using a hand blender with a whisk connection, beat the egg whites until medium-firm pinnacles structure. They ought to scarcely move in the event that you tilt the bowl and ought not to spill out.

3.   Gradually include the sugar, 1-2 tablespoons (14 grams) one after another, while beating continually. Beat in the ocean salt and vanilla concentrate.

4.   Gently overlay in the coconut pieces, being mindful so as not to separate the whites.

5.   Use medium scoop to drop the hitter onto the lined container.

6.   Bake for 15 to 20 minutes, until brilliant dark-colored.

7.   Make the discretionary chocolate shower: In the microwave or a twofold evaporator on the stove, liquefy the chocolate chips and coconut oil, blending until smooth. Sprinkle the chocolate on the macaroons.

8.
Cool the macaroons until no longer hot; at that point, refrigerate for around 20 to 30 minutes to set the chocolate.

Formula NOTES

Serving size: 1 macaroon cookie

NUTRITION INFORMATION PER SERVING

Nutrition Facts

Sum per serving. Serving size in formula notes above.

Calories135

Fat11g

Protein1g

Absolute Carbs5g

Net Carbs2g

Fiber3g

Sugar1g

21. LOW CARB GLUTEN-FREE GINGER SNAPS COOKIES RECIPE

This without gluten ginger snaps formula suggests a flavor like the genuine article! You just need 6 fixings and one bowl to make these simple low carb ginger snaps cookies.

Course Dessert

.

Calories 140 kcal

Planning Time 10 minutes

Cook Time 15 minutes

Absolute Time 25 minutes

Servings 2" cookies

This can't be played

Fixings

 6 tbsp Butter (relaxed; can utilize coconut oil for sans dairy, yet flavor and surface will be extraordinary)

  1/3 cup Golden priest organic product sugar mix

  2 tsp Cinnamon

  1/2 tbsp ground ginger

  1/4 tsp Sea salt

  1 tsp Vanilla concentrate

  2 1/2 cups Blanched almond flour

Guidelines

1. Preheat the broiler to 350 degrees F (177 degrees C). Line a heating sheet with material paper.

2. Using a hand blender at medium speed, cream margarine, and sugar together until feathery.

3. Beat in the cinnamon, ginger, ocean salt, and vanilla concentrate.

4. Beat the almond flour, 1/2 cup (64 g) at once.

5. Use a medium cookie scoop to scoop the mixture and press it into the scoop. Discharge onto the lined heating sheet and straighten utilizing your palm. Orchestrate cookies in any event 1.5 inches (4 cm) separated.

6. Bake for about 15 to 20 minutes. Cool totally before moving. Cookies will fresh up as they cool.

Formula NOTES

Serving size: 1 2-inch cookie

NUTRITION INFORMATION PER SERVING

Nutrition Facts

Sum per serving. Serving size in formula notes above.

Calories140

Fat13g

Protein3g

All out Carbs4g

Net Carbs2g

Fiber2g

Sugar0g

22. THE MOST FUDGY KETO BROWNIES RECIPE - 6 INGREDIENTS

The BEST keto brownies formula, prepared in less than 30 minutes! Only 6 fixings expected to make simple fudgy keto brownies with almond flour.

Course Dessert

.

Calories 174 kcal

Planning Time 10 minutes

Cook Time 15 minutes

All out Time 25 minutes

Servings brownies

Fixings

> 1/2 cup butter

> 4 oz Unsweetened heating chocolate

> 3/4 cup Blanched almond flour

> 2/3 cup Powdered allulose (or powdered erythritol)

> 2 tbsp Cocoa powder

> 2 enormous Eggs (at room temperature)

> 1 tsp Vanilla concentrate (discretionary)

> 1/4 tsp Sea salt (just if utilizing unsalted spread)

> 1/4 cup Walnuts (discretionary, cleaved)

Guidelines

1.   Preheat the broiler to 350 degrees F (177 degrees C). Line an 8x8 in (20x20 cm) skillet with material paper, with the edges of the paper over the sides.

2.   Melt the margarine and chocolate altogether in a twofold evaporator, blending once in a while, until smooth. Expel from heat.

3.   Stir in the vanilla concentrate.

4.   Add the almond flour, powdered sugar, cocoa powder, ocean salt, and eggs. Mix together until uniform. The hitter will be somewhat grainy looking.

5.   Transfer the hitter to the lined dish. Smooth the top of the spatula or the rear of a spoon. Whenever wanted, sprinkle with cleaved pecans and press into the top.

6.   Bake for around 13-18 minutes until an embedded toothpick tells the truth with only a little hitter on it that balls up between your fingers. (Try not to hang tight for it to confess all, and don't stress over any margarine pooled on top - simply watch the genuine brownie part to be excessively delicate however not liquid.)

7.   Cool totally before moving or cutting. There might be some spread pooled on top - don't deplete it, it will retain back in the wake of cooling.

Formula NOTES

Serving size: 1 brownie (1/16 of whole formula)

Update: This formula was initially composed of 3/4 cup spread and utilizing granulated erythritol. It has been refreshed to 1/2 cup spread and using powdered sugar rather, which in testing has made better outcomes (more fudgy brownies). The variant in my cookbook utilizes powdered erythritol and the adaptation above utilizations powdered allulose, which makes even smoother fudge brownies. This data is here in the event that you favor one of the old adaptations.

Nutrition information does exclude discretionary pecans.

NUTRITION INFORMATION PER SERVING

Nutrition Facts

Sum per serving. Serving size in formula notes above.

Calories174

Fat16g

Protein3g

Absolute Carbs4g

Net Carbs2g

Fiber2g

Sugar0g

23. THE BEST KETO SUGAR-FREE PECAN PIE RECIPE

This keto walnut pie formula is the just a single you'll ever requirement for the best sans sugar walnut pie ever! Simple to make and simply like the genuine article.

Course Dessert

.

Calories 533 kcal

Planning Time 5 minutes

Cook Time 60 minutes

Cooling Time 15 minutes

All out Time 1 hour 20 minutes

Servings cuts

Fixings

1 formula Almond flour pie outside layer (or coconut flour pie covering)

3/4 cup of Butter

3/4 cup of Besti Powdered Monk Fruit Erythritol Blend (or priest organic product allulose mix for a gooey walnut pie)

1 1/2 cup Heavy cream

1 tsp Sea salt

1/2 tbsp Vanilla concentrate

3/4 tsp Maple separate

1 enormous Egg (at room temperature)

2 1/2 cups Pecans (2 cups slashed coarsely + 1/2 cup parts for garnish)

Guidelines

Preheat the broiler to 350 degrees F (177 degrees C).

1.   Make the almond flour pie outside layer, as indicated by the guidelines here.

2.   Meanwhile, make the filling. In an enormous saute skillet (not a pan!) over medium-low warmth, heat the margarine and sugar for around 5 minutes, regularly blending, until dull brilliant dark-colored.

3.   When brilliant, include the cream and ocean salt. Bring to a delicate stew. Stew for 15 to 20 minutes, until bubbly, dull brilliant and thick. The caramel sauce should cover the rear of a spoon.

4.   Remove the sauce from heat. Mix in the vanilla and maple separates.

5.   Let pie outside layer and caramel sauce cool independently for 15 to 20 minutes, until warm yet not hot. While cooling, you can either leave the broiler on (you will require it once more.

6.   Once the caramel sauce has cooled enough not to cook an egg being added to it (warm is fine), race in the egg.

7.   Place slashed walnuts equally into the outside layer. Pour the caramel/egg blend over the walnuts. Top with walnut parts.

8.   Cover the edges of the pie outside layer with foil, leaving the middle open.

9.   Bake for around 40 to 50 minutes until the top is dim dark-colored, and the filling is set, aside from certain air pockets on the top.

10.   Cool totally, at that point, chill for at any rate an hour prior to cutting.

Formula NOTES

Serving size: 1 cut, or 1/12 of the whole pie

NUTRITION INFORMATION PER SERVING

Nutrition Facts

Sum per serving. Serving size in formula notes above.

Calories533

Fat54g

Protein9g

Complete Carbs8g

Net Carbs4g

Fiber4g

Sugar2g

24. LOW CARB KETO CHOCOLATE BAR RECIPE

Figure out how to make low carb chocolate bars! This is the ideal approach to make a keto chocolate bar that suggests a flavor like the genuine article. Incorporates which sugars to utilize and the best strategy.

Course Dessert

.

Calories 143 kcal

Planning Time 5 minutes

Cook Time 5 minutes

Refrigerate 30 minutes

All out Time 10 minutes

Servings

Fixings

> 3 oz Cocoa margarine or 2 tbsp coconut oil, however, will be more liquefy.
>
> 2 1/2 oz Unsweetened heating chocolate
>
> 6 tbsp Powdered erythritol
>
> 2 tbsp Inulin
>
> 1/4 tsp Liquid sunflower lecithin
>
> 1/8 tsp Sea salt
>
> 1 tsp Vanilla concentrate

Guidelines

1.   Melt cocoa margarine and preparing chocolate in a twofold evaporator over low warmth.

2.   Stir in the powdered erythritol, a little at once. Mix in the inulin, a little at once. Mix in the sunflower lecithin and salt. Warmth until everything is smooth and broke up.

3.   Remove from heat. Mix in vanilla concentrate.

4.   Pour the liquefied chocolate blend into molds. Refrigerate for at any rate 30 minutes, until firm.

Formula NOTES

Serving size: 6 squares, or 1/4 of a chocolate bar

•   Recipe makes 2 standard-size chocolate bars.

NUTRITION INFORMATION PER SERVING

Nutrition Facts

Sum per serving. Serving size in formula notes above.

Calories143

Fat15g

Protein1g

All out Carbs4g

Net Carbs1g

Fiber3g

Sugar0g

25. LOW CARB KETO PUMPKIN CHEESECAKE RECIPE

An unimaginably smooth, tap keto pumpkin cheesecake! This simple low carb pumpkin cheesecake formula could possibly turn into your preferred low carb pumpkin dessert ever.

Course Dessert

.

Calories 280 kcal

Planning Time 15 minutes

Cook Time 55 minutes

Absolute Time 1 hour 10 minutes

Servings cuts

Fixings

Almond Flour Cheesecake Crust

   1 1/2 cup Blanched almond flour

   1/2 cup Vital Proteins Collagen Peptides (or whey protein powder)

   3 tbsp Allulose

   1/3 cup Butter (dissolved)

   1 tsp Vanilla concentrate

Pumpkin Cheesecake Filling

   24 oz Cream cheddar (mollified)

   1 cup pumpkin puree

   1 1/4 cup Powdered allulose

   3 huge eggs (at room temperature)

   1 tsp Pumpkin pie flavor

   1/2 tsp Cinnamon

   1 tsp Vanilla concentrate

Directions

1.   Preheat the cooker to 350 degrees F (177 degrees C). Line the base of a 9 in (23 cm) springform container with material paper. (You can likewise have a go at lubing great.)

2.   To make the almond flour cheesecake outside, mix the almond flour, collagen or protein powder, and sugar together.

3.   Whisk together the liquefied spread and vanilla, at that point mix into the dry fixings, squeezing with the spoon or spatula, until all around joined. The mixture will be somewhat brittle.

4.   Press the batter into the base of the readied container. Prick delicately with a fork everywhere. Heat for around 12-15 minutes, until scarcely brilliant. Let cool at any rate of 10 minutes.

5.   Meanwhile, beat the cream cheddar and powdered sugar together at low to medium speed until cushioned. Beat in the pumpkin puree, pumpkin pie zest, cinnamon, and vanilla. Beat in the eggs, each in turn. (Keep the blender at low to medium the entire time; too rapid will present too many air bubbles, which we don't need.)

6.   Pour the filling into the container over the outside. Smooth the top with a spatula. (Utilize a cake spatula for a smoother top in the event that you have one that fits into the skillet.)

7.   Bake for around 40-50 minutes, until the inside is nearly set, yet jiggly.

8.   Remove the cheesecake from the broiler. In the event that the edges adhere to the dish, run a blade around the edge. (In any case, don't expel the springform edge at this time.) Cool the cheesecake in the skillet on the counter to room temperature, at that point refrigerate for in any event 4 hours (ideally medium-term), until totally set. (Try not to attempt to expel the cake from the container before chilling.)

9.   Serve with whipped cream as well as a sprinkle of cinnamon.

Formula NOTES

Serving size: 1 cut (1/16 of formula)

*This formula was initially made utilizing erythritol for the hull and powdered erythritol for the filling, yet has been refreshed to utilize allulose and powdered allulose, separately, for a better surface.

NUTRITION INFORMATION PER SERVING

Nutrition Facts

Sum per serving. Serving size in formula notes above.

Calories280

Fat24g

Protein10g

Complete Carbs6g

Net Carbs5g

Fiber1g

Sugar2g

26. Simple KETO FUDGE RECIPE WITH COCOA POWDER and SEA SALT

This simple keto fudge formula needs only 4 fixings and 10 minutes prep! Also, making keto fudge with cocoa powder and ocean salt is excessively simple.

Course Dessert

.

Calories 161 kcal

Planning Time 10 minutes

Cook Time 45 minutes

Aloof Time 45 minutes

All out Time 55 minutes

Servings

Fixings

     1 cup Coconut oil (strong)

     1/4 cup Powdered erythritol (to taste)

     1/4 cup Cocoa powder

     1 tsp Vanilla concentrate

     1/8 tsp Sea salt

     Coarse ocean salt drops (discretionary - for fixing)

Guidelines

1.   Line a 28 oz rectangular glass holder with material paper, so the material hangs out over the sides.

2.   Using a hand blender at LOW speed, beat the coconut oil and sugar together, just until soft and joined.

3.   Beat in the cocoa powder, vanilla, and ocean salt to taste. Modify sugar to taste. Don't overmix.

4.   Transfer the blend to the lined holder. Strai the top with a spatula or spoon.

5.   Refrigerate the keto fudge for around 45-an hour, until strong.

6.   Sprinkle the highest point of the fudge with ocean salt pieces and press delicately.

7.   Run a blade along the edge and take out utilizing the edges of the material paper. Cut cautiously - see post above for cutting tips.

8.   Keep the fudge refrigerated and bring it to room temperature directly before serving. You can likewise freeze it - see tips above. Try not to leave at room temperature for delayed periods, as it will liquefy no problem at all.

Formula NOTES

Serving size: 1 3D shape, or 1/12 of the whole formula

NUTRITION INFORMATION PER SERVING

Nutrition Facts

Sum per serving. Serving size in formula notes above.

Calories161

Fat18g

Protein0g

Absolute Carbs1g

Net Carbs0.4g

Fiber0.6g

Sugar02

LOW CARB DOUBLE CHOCOLATE PROTEIN MUFFINS RECIPE

These low carb twofold chocolate protein biscuits are anything but difficult to make, damp, and tasty. This healthy protein biscuit formula needs only 10 minutes of planning time!

Course Breakfast, Dessert

.

Calories 233 kcal

Planning Time 10 minutes

Cook Time 25 minutes

All out Time 35 minutes

Servings biscuits

This can't be played

Fixings

   2 cup Blanched almond flour

   2/3 cup Allulose (or any granulated sugar)

   1/2 cup Cocoa powder

   1/4 cup Vital Proteins Collagen Peptides

   1 1/2 tsp without gluten preparing powder

   1/4 tsp Sea salt

   1/3 cup Coconut oil

   1/2 cup unsweetened almond milk

   3 huge Eggs

   1/2 tsp Vanilla concentrate

   3/4 cup without sugar dull chocolate chips

Directions

1.   Preheat the cooker to 350 degrees F (177 degrees C). Line a biscuit dish with 12 material paper liners or silicone biscuit liners.

2.   In a huge bowl, mix together the almond flour, sugar, cocoa powder, collagen peptides, preparing powder, and ocean salt.

3.   Stir in the dissolved coconut oil and almond milk. Rush in the eggs and vanilla. Crease in the chocolate chips last. (On the off chance that you'd like, you can save 1/4 cup of the chocolate chips to add on top.)

4.   Scoop the hitter equitably into the biscuit cups, filling practically full. On the off chance that you saved some chocolate contributes the past advance, sprinkle them on top, and press delicately into the player.

5.   Bake for about 25 titles, until the tops are brilliant and an embedded toothpick confesses all.

Formula NOTES

Serving size: 1 biscuit

NUTRITION INFORMATION PER SERVING

Nutrition Facts

Sum per serving. Serving size in formula notes above.

Calories233

Fat20g

Protein10g

All out Carbs10g

Net Carbs5g

Fiber5g

Sugar0g

27. CHOCOLATE CHIP LOW CARB PALEO ZUCCHINI OF MUFFINS RECIPE

For the most heavenly low carb zucchini biscuits or paleo zucchini biscuits, attempt this chocolate chip zucchini biscuits formula with coconut flour! It's without sugar, keto, sans nut, and sans dairy.

Course Breakfast, Dessert

.

Calories 181 kcal

Planning Time 10 minutes

Cook Time 35 minutes

All out Time 45 minutes

Servings biscuits

Fixings

   3/4 cup Coconut flour

   1/2 cup Erythritol

   2 tsp sans gluten heating powder

   1/4 tsp Sea salt

   8 oz Zucchini (destroyed/ground, around 2 cups)

   6 enormous Egg

   1/2 tsp Vanilla concentrate

   2/3 cup Ghee (estimated strong, at that point softened; can likewise utilize sans dairy spread enhanced coconut oil)

   1/2 cup sans sugar dim chocolate chips

Guidelines

1.   Preheat the broiler to 350 degrees F (177 degrees C). Line a biscuit container with 12 material paper liners.

2.   In an enormous bowl, mix together the coconut flour, sugar, heating powder, and ocean salt.

3.   Add the destroyed zucchini, eggs, and vanilla. Mix together until joined. Include the liquefied coconut oil and mix again until smooth.

4.   Fold in the chocolate chips. Let the player sit for 5 minutes to thicken.

5.   Divide the hitter among the material liners, filling them right to the top. Whenever wanted, you can spot the tops with more chocolate chips.

6.   Bake for around 35 minutes, until brilliant and firm on top. Cool to room temperature in the dish, at that point on a wire rack. You can eat them warm; however, the surface is better in the event that you let them cool first.

Formula NOTES

Serving size: 1 biscuit

NUTRITION INFORMATION PER SERVING

Nutrition Facts

Sum per serving. Serving size in formula notes above.

Calories181

Fat15g

Protein5g

Complete Carbs8g

Net Carbs4g

Fiber4g

Sugar1g

28. LOW CARB CHOCOLATE CHIP PEANUT BUTTER OF PROTEIN COOKIES RECIPE

This simple chocolate chip peanut spread protein cookies formula is so chewy! Only 6 fixings, 1 bowl, and 10 minutes prep for tasty, flourless low carb protein cookies. They're normally sans gluten.

Course Breakfast, Dessert

.

Calories 118 kcal

Planning Time 10 minutes

Cook Time 20 minutes

Complete Time 30 minutes

Servings cookies

Fixings

    1/3 cup Vital Proteins Collagen Peptides

    1/2 cup Erythritol (or any granulated sugar)

    1/4 tsp Sea salt

    1 cup Peanut margarine (no sugar included)

    2 enormous Eggs

    1 tsp Vanilla concentrate

    1/3 cup sans sugar dim chocolate chips

Guidelines

1.   Preheat the broiler to 350 degrees F (177 degrees C). Line a heating sheet with material paper.

2.   In an enormous bowl, mix together the collagen, sugar, and ocean salt.

3.   Add the egg and race at the edge of the bowl to blend the yolk and white, before blending in with the dry fixings. Include the peanut margarine and vanilla, and mix until smooth.

4.   Fold in the chocolate chips.

5.   Scoop the cookie mixture utilizing a medium cookie scoop and press the batter into it before discharging onto the lined heating sheet. Squash the cookie batter balls with the palm of your hand or the base of a wet glass, to around 1/4 in (~1/2 cm) thickness.

6.   Bake for around 16-20 minutes, until the cookies are semi-firm and not clingy on top. Cool totally to solidify more.

Formula NOTES

Serving size: 1 cookie

NUTRITION INFORMATION PER SERVING

Nutrition Facts

Sum per serving. Serving size in formula notes above.

Calories118

Fat8g

Protein7g

Absolute Carbs4g

Net Carbs2g

Fiber2g

Sugar0g

29. HEALTHY SUGAR-FREE LOW CARB BLACKBERRY COBBLER RECIPE

This simple without sugar blackberry shoemaker formula needs only 10 minutes prep! So delightful, nobody will realize this is a low carb blackberry shoemaker.

Course Dessert

.

Calories 154 kcal

Planning Time 10 minutes

Cook Time 25 minutes

Absolute Time 35 minutes

Servings

This can't be played

Fixings

Blackberry Cobbler Filling

    1 lb Blackberries

    2 tbsp Lemon juice

    1/3 cup of Besti Monk Fruit Allulose Blend (or 1/4 cup on the off chance that you need it less sweet)

    2 tbsp Vital Proteins Grass-took care of Gelatin

Shoemaker Topping

    1 cup Blanched almond flour

    1/4 cup Besti Monk Fruit Allulose Blend (or 3 tbsp on the off chance that you need it less sweet)

    1/2 tsp sans gluten preparing powder

    1/4 tsp Sea salt

    1/4 cup Coconut oil (can likewise utilize margarine or ghee if not without dairy)

    1/2 tsp Vanilla concentrate

Guidelines

1.   Preheat the broiler to 350 degrees F.

2.   In an enormous bowl, hurl together the berries, lemon juice, and sugar. Sprinkle (don't dump) tablespoon gelatin over the blend and blend to join, at that point, rehash with the other tablespoon gelatin.

3.   Transfer the berries to the base of a glass or non-stick 8x8 inch (20x20 cm) heating container.

4.   In another enormous bowl in the microwave or a pan on the stove, dissolve the coconut oil. Expel from heat.

5.   Stir the vanilla concentrate into the softened coconut oil. Mix in the almond flour, sugar, heating powder, and ocean salt. The batter ought to be brittle, yet rich and somewhat clammy.

6.   Crumble the mixture over the highest point of the berries in the dish, leaving some little spaces of berries radiating through.

7.   Bake the shoemaker for around 25-30 minutes, until the top is brilliant. Rest at any rate 10 minutes before serving, or cool to room temperature for considerably thicker shoemaker.

Formula NOTES

Serving size: 1/9 of the whole formula

On the off chance that you serve the shoemaker in 3 squares by squares toward every path, a serving is a 2.5x2.5" square.

NUTRITION INFORMATION PER SERVING

Nutrition Facts

Sum per serving. Serving size in formula notes above.

Calories154

Fat12g

Protein5g

All out Carbs7g

Net Carbs3g

Fiber4g

Sugar3g

30. ATKINS ICE OF CREAM RECIPE WITHOUT ICE CREAM MAKER

You just need 4 fixings and 20 minutes prep to make this simple Atkins dessert formula without a frozen yogurt producer! Appreciate protein-rich dessert without sugar.

Course Dessert

.

Calories 190 kcal

Planning Time 10 minutes

Cook Time 10 minutes

Freezing time 4 hours

Complete Time 4 hours 40 minutes

Servings

Fixings

1 11-oz container Atkins Plus Protein and Fiber Creamy Vanilla Shake

1 1/2 cup of heavy cream

1/4 cup of powdered erythritol (or any powdered sugar of decision)

2 huge Egg

Directions

Make custard

1.   Separate the eggs first into two huge dishes. Put in a safe spot.

2.   Combine the shake, overwhelming cream, and sugar in an enormous pot. Warmth over medium warmth for a couple of moments, mixing at times, until rising close to the edges.

3.   Mix together the yolks in the bowl where you isolated them. Gradually empty the cream blend into the egg yolks in a slender stream, whisking continually. (To do this way to "temper.")

4.   Return the blend to the pan. Warmth delicately while mixing continually for a couple of moments, until the blend scarcely covers the rear of a spoon. It won't be as thick as a customary custard.

5.   Remove from warm and empty the blend once again into the bowl where the yolks began. Spread flush against the top with material paper to keep a film from framing. Chill for 60 minutes.

Overlap custard into whipped egg whites

1.   In the bowl where you had set the egg whites, utilize a hand blender to whip them until firm pinnacles structure. (They will be room temperature at this point, which is the thing that you need.)

2.   Remove the custard blend from the ice chest and whisk once more. In the event that there is any film on the top, skim it off.

3.   Fold the blend into the egg whites, until uniform. The whites will fall, yet the final product will, in any case, be somewhat more fleecy than simply fluid.

Freeze

1.   Freeze as per frozen yogurt creator directions.

2.   If you don't have a frozen yogurt producer, tenderly empty the blend into a glass or material lined safe cooler compartment. Freeze for 4-5 hours, collapsing the blend delicately to separate precious ice stones at regular intervals for the initial 2 hours. In the event that frozen yogurt turns out to be too hard after quite a while, defrost on the counter before serving.

Formula NOTES

Serving size: 1/2 cup

NUTRITION INFORMATION PER SERVING

Nutrition Facts

Sum per serving. Serving size in formula notes above.

Calories190

Fat18g

Protein4g

Complete Carbs1g

Net Carbs1g

Fiber0g

Sugar1g

31. GLUTEN-FREE SUGAR-FREE STRAWBERRY PIE RECIPE WITH GELATIN

Make this simple sans gluten strawberry pie formula with crisp or solidified strawberries. Only 5 fixings, in addition to coconut flour hull! Sans sugar strawberry pie is low carb, keto, and has a paleo alternative.

Course Dessert

.

Calories 144 kcal

Planning Time 10 minutes

Cook Time 20 minutes

Complete Time 30 minutes

Servings cuts

Fixings

    1 formula Coconut flour pie outside layer (or any covering you like)

    2 lb Strawberries (crisp or solidified)

    1 cup Powdered erythritol (or any sugar of decision)

    3 tbsp Vital Proteins Grass-Fed Gelatin

    1/2 cup Water

    2 tbsp Lemon juice

Guidelines

1.   Bake the coconut flour pie outside layer, as indicated by the guidelines here.

2.   Meanwhile, in an enormous pot over medium warmth, stew the strawberries with powdered erythritol for around 15 minutes, until strawberries are delicate. Mix once in a while.

3.   While strawberries stew, whisk together the gelatin, water, and lemon squeeze in a little bowl.

4.   Whisk the gelatin blend into the strawberries. Stew for two or three minutes, blending/speeding until the gelatin breaks down.

5.   Let the strawberry filling and pie hull cool independently for 20 minutes.

6.   Put the strawberry filling into the prepared pie covering. Cool on the counter, at that point, refrigerate medium-term .to set. Enhancement with whipped cream and crisp strawberries to serve.

Formula NOTES

Serving size: 1 cut, or 1/12 of the whole formula

NUTRITION INFORMATION PER SERVING

Nutrition Facts

Sum per serving. Serving size in formula notes above.

Calories144

Fat9g

Protein4g

Complete Carbs9g

Net Carbs6g

Fiber3g

Sugar3g

32. THE COCONUT FLOUR PIE & THE CRUST RECIPE

It's overly simple to figure out how to make pie outside layer with coconut flour! This simple coconut flour pie outside layer formula is low carb, keto, without gluten, rich and tasty. Just 5 fixings!

Course Dessert

.

Calories 111 kcal

Planning Time 10 minutes

Cook Time 10 minutes

Absolute Time 20 minutes

Servings cuts

Fixings

3/4 cup of oconut flour

1/2 cup of butter (cool, cut into pieces)

1/3 cup of erythritol (skip for exquisite hull)

1/4 tsp of sea salt (or 1/2 tsp for appetizing outside layer)

2 huge Egg

1/2 tsp Vanilla concentrate (discretionary, skip for appetizing outside layer)

Directions

1.   Preheat the cooker to 350 degrees F (177 degrees C). Line the base of a 9 in (23 cm) round pie dish with material paper, or oil well.

2.   Combine the coconut flour, spread, erythritol, and ocean salt in a food processor. Heartbeat until all around consolidated.

3.   Add the eggs and vanilla concentrate. Procedure again until batter structures.

4.   Press the coconut flour pie outside layer batter into the pie dish. Jab gaps in the base with a fork or toothpick.

5.   Bake for 10-15 minutes, until firm and marginally brilliant on the edges. Lay on the counter for in any event 10 minutes before including filling; at that point, you can prepare again varying for the filling. In the event that the edges begin to dark-colored a lot before the filling is done, you can cover them with foil. Cool totally before cutting.

Formula NOTES

Serving size: 1 cut, or 1/12 of the whole formula

NUTRITION INFORMATION PER SERVING

Nutrition Facts

Sum per serving. Serving size in formula notes above.

Calories111

Fat9g

Protein2g

Complete Carbs4g

Net Carbs2g

Fiber2g

Sugar0g

33. CHOCOLATE PEANUT BUTTER OF NICE CREAM RECIPE - 5 INGREDIENTS

Figure out how to make decent cream without bananas or a dessert creator! This delectable chocolate peanut spread pleasant cream formula is without sugar, low carb, keto, and veggie lover. Only 5 fixings and 5 minutes of planning time!

Course Dessert

.

Calories 362 kcal

Planning Time 5 minutes

Latent Time 3 hours

All out Time 3 hours 5 minutes

Servings

Fixings

    1 13.5-oz would coconut be able to drain (full-fat)

    1/2 cup Peanut margarine (rich, no sugar included)

    1/3 cup Coconut oil (estimated strong, at that point liquefied)

    1/4 cup of Cocoa powder

    1/2 cup of Powdered allulose (or any powdered sweetener*)

    1 squeeze Sea salt (discretionary - to taste)

Guidelines

1.   Puree all fixings in an amazing blender or food processor, until smooth.

2.   Pour the blend into a 1/2 or 2 quart (2 liters) glass cooler safe holder. Spread and freeze for 30 minutes, at that point mix well, particularly mixing ceaselessly from the sides into the middle. Spread and freeze for 30 additional minutes and mix once more. Spread and freeze for 2-3 additional hours, until firm.

3.   Chocolate peanut spread pleasant cream is the best consistency in the wake of freezing for 3-4 hours. In the case of putting away for more, essentially defrost on the counter for about an hour to mellow before eating.

Formula NOTES

Serving size: 1/2 cup

*Other powdered sugars will work, yet I suggest allulose for scoop-capable frozen yogurt that doesn't get excessively hard in the cooler.

NUTRITION INFORMATION PER SERVING

Nutrition Facts

Sum per serving. Serving size in formula notes above.

Calories362

Fat35g

Protein6g

All out Carbs8g

Net Carbs5g

Fiber3g

Sugar1g

34. FATHEAD KETO CINNAMON ROLLS RECIPE - QUICK and EASY

Everybody adores these keto cinnamon rolls! Just 40 minutes to make, with straightforward fixings (no uncommon flour!), and they're absolutely tasty. For an astonishing low carb dessert or keto breakfast, attempt this fathead cinnamon moves formula.

Course Breakfast, Dessert

Calories 321 kcal

Planning Time 20 minutes

Cook Time 20 minutes

Complete Time 40 minutes

Servings cinnamon rolls

Fixings

   2 cup Macadamia nuts (10 oz)

   1/4 cup Erythritol

   1 tbsp sans gluten heating powder

   2 enormous Egg

   1 tsp Vanilla concentrate (discretionary)

   4 cup Mozzarella cheddar (destroyed)

   4 oz Cream cheddar

Filling

   1/4 cup butter (softened)

   1/2 cup Erythritol

   2 tbsp Cinnamon

Icing

   1/3 cup sans sugar cream cheddar icing

   1 tbsp of unsweetened almond milk (or any milk of decision)

Guidelines

1.   Put the macadamia nuts into a food processor fitted with a blade cutting edge. Heartbeat just until the nuts arrive at a fine, brittle consistency, without huge pieces. Make a point to beat, don't leave the food processor running, to attempt to make flour and not nut margarine. Scratch the sides varying. The nuts may, in any case, start to shape nut spread a bit, however, attempt to dodge however much as could be expected.

2.   Add the erythritol and heating powder. Heartbeat two or multiple times, just until blended.

3.   Add the eggs and vanilla. Heartbeat a few times once more, just until blended.

4.   Heat the mozzarella and cream cheddar in the microwave for around 2 minutes, mixing partially through and toward the end, or on the stove in a twofold heater, until simple to mix. Mix until smooth.

5.   Add the cheddar blend to the food processor. Push the cheddar blend down into the nut/egg blend. Heartbeat/puree until a uniform batter structure, scratching down the sides vary. If at all you experience difficulty getting it to blend, you can manipulate a little with a spatula and afterward beat some more.

6.   Refrigerate the mixture directly in the food processor for around 30-an hour, until the top is firm and not clingy.

7.   Meanwhile, preheat the broiler to 375 degrees F (191 degrees C). Line a 9x13 in (23x33 cm) heating dish with material paper.

8.   Take the mixture out onto an enormous bit of material paper (not the one on the preparing sheet). It will at present, be genuinely clingy. Utilize a smidgen of the softened margarine on your hands to forestall staying as you spread it into a square shape. Spot another bit of material on top and turn out to a more slender square shape, around 14 in (36 cm) long by 10 in (25 cm) wide with 1/3 to 1/2 of (8 to 13 mm) thick.

9.   Brush the mixture square shape with the vast majority of the staying dissolved margarine, leaving aside around 1-2 tablespoons. Mix together the erythritol and cinnamon for the filling. Sprinkle the blend equitably over the square shape.

10.   Oil your hands again with the dissolved margarine. Beginning from a long side of the square shape, fold up the batter into a log. As you come, oil the underside of the log as you strip it away from the material underneath during rolling. (This is to forestall breaking and staying.)

11.   Slice the sign into 1 in (2.5 cm) thick cuts, which will look like pinwheels. Spot the pinwheels level onto the lined preparing container, practically contacting yet not exactly.

12.   Bake for around 25 minutes, until the keto cinnamon rolls are brilliant on top. Cool for in any event 20 minutes, until firm.

13.	Meanwhile, making the icing. Beat almond milk into the icing a tablespoon at once, until the icing is sufficiently slight to shower. When the keto cinnamon rolls are sufficiently firm, sprinkle the icing over them.

Formula NOTES

Serving size: 1 cinnamon roll

NUTRITION INFORMATION PER SERVING

Nutrition Facts

Sum per serving. Serving size in formula notes above.

Calories321

Fat29.5g

Protein11g

Absolute Carbs5g

Net Carbs3g

Fiber2g

Sugar1g

35. THE EASY CHOCOLATE FAT BOMBS WITH COCONUT OIL

. These simple, ketogenic chocolate fat bombs with coconut oil, MCT oil, and macadamia nuts taste unbelievable and are ideal for a low carb, paleo, or ketogenic diet.

Course Dessert, Snack

.

Calories 122 kcal

Planning Time 10 minutes

Complete Time 10 minutes

Servings fat bombs

Fixings

2 cup Macadamia nuts (dry simmered, salted)

2 tbsp Coconut oil (estimated strong, at that point softened)

2 tbsp of MCT oil (or more coconut oil for firmer fat bombs)

1 tsp of Vanilla concentrate (discretionary)

1/3 cup of Besti Powdered Monk Fruit Allulose Blend

1/4 cup of Cocoa powder

Guidelines

1.   Pure macadamia nuts into a food processor or high force blender, until generally separated into little pieces. Include MCT oil, liquefied coconut oil, and vanilla. Keep on pureeing until nut margarine structures. (Attempt to get it smooth, yet on the off chance that you can't dispose of some wanderer pieces, that is alright!) Scrape down the sides as vital.

2.   Add the cocoa powder and sugar step by step, two or three tablespoons one after another. Puree after every expansion, until smooth.

3.   Line a smaller than normal biscuit dish with material liners. Pour or spoon the player uniformly into every liner, around 1/3 of the way full.

4.   Freeze for at any rate 30 minutes, until strong.

Formula NOTES

Utilize salted macadamia nuts. On the off chance that yours are unsalted, add some ocean salt to taste.

Serving size: 1 fat bomb

NUTRITION INFORMATION PER SERVING

Nutrition Facts

Sum per serving. Serving size in formula notes above.

Calories122

Fat13g

Protein1g

All out Carbs2g

Net Carbs1g

Fiber1g

Sugar0g

36. GLUTEN-FREE SUGAR-FREE FLOURLESS CHOCOLATE CAKE RECIPE

This sans gluten sans sugar flourless chocolate cake formula needs only FIVE INGREDIENTS! Made with sans sugar chocolate and your sugar of decision, this is the best flourless chocolate cake formula ever! Normally keto and low carb.

Course Dessert

.

Calories 349 kcal

Planning Time 10 minutes

Cook Time 30 minutes

Complete Time 40 minutes

Servings cuts

Fixings

   1 1/2 cup Butter

   24 oz without sugar dull chocolate (cleaved; use sans sugar, not unsweetened!)

   1 1/2 tsp Vanilla concentrate

   1/4 tsp Sea salt (discretionary - skip if utilizing salted spread)

   6 huge Egg (at room temperature)

   1/2 cup Besti Powdered Monk Fruit Allulose Blend

Directions

1.   Preheat the Cooker to 350 degrees F (177 degrees C). Line the base of a 9 in (23 cm) springform skillet with material paper. Oil the base and sides.

2.   Melt the chocolate and spread together, in a twofold heater on the stove or at medium-low force in the microwave, blending infrequently. Try not to overheat to abstain from parting.

3.   Remove from warm and empty the chocolate blend into an enormous bowl. Utilize a hand blender to beat in the vanilla and ocean salt at *low* speed.

4.   Beat in the eggs at *low* speed, each in turn.

5.   Beat in the powdered sugar, still at low speed. The blend ought to be to some degree smooth, yet somewhat uneven.

6.   Pour the player into the lined dish. Smooth the top with a spatula. Spot the springform container onto a preparing sheet to get any releases, in the event that something goes wrong.

7.   Bake for 25 min. till the top just begins to shape a slight outside layer on the edges just, and the inner temperature in the inside by means of thermometer is 140 degrees F (60 degrees C). The cake won't look done, which is typical, so pass by the temperature.

8.   Cool to room temperature in the skillet, at that point refrigerate medium-term (at any rate 8 hours) directly in the container.

9.   Remove the skillet from the ice chest 1 hour before serving. Fly off the sides of the springform container and move to a plate or cake stand. Residue with extra powdered sugar whenever wanted. Let the cake arrive at room temperature before cutting.

Formula NOTES

Serving size: 1 cut, or 1/16 of the whole flourless chocolate cake

•   Make sure to utilize without sugar stevia improved chocolate like this, not unsweetened pastry specialist's chocolate!

•   This formula was initially made utilizing powdered erythritol, however now I enthusiastically suggest Besti Powdered Monk Fruit Allulose Blend for the best surface.

NUTRITION INFORMATION PER SERVING

Nutrition Facts

Sum per serving. Serving size in formula notes above.

Calories349

Fat34g

Protein4g

All out Carbs17g

Net Carbs5g

Fiber12g

Sugar0g

37. LOW CARB KETO PROTEIN COOKIE DOUGH BITES RECIPE

Perceive how to make natively constructed palatable cookie mixture that is sans gluten and without sugar! These low carb keto protein cookie batter chomps are flavorful, healthy, and EASY.

Course Appetizer, Dessert, Snack

.

Calories 169 kcal

Planning Time 10 minutes

All out Time 30 minutes

Servings (2 1" nibbles each)

Fixings

    1/2 cup Butter (relaxed; or coconut oil for sans dairy)

    1/3 cup Powdered erythritol (or more to taste)

    1 tsp Vanilla concentrate

    1/4 tsp blackstrap molasses (discretionary, prescribed for cookie mixture season)

     1/4 cup of Blanched almond flour (or sunflower seed meal for sans nut)

    1/2 cup Vital Proteins Vanilla Collagen Peptides

    1/4 tsp Sea salt

    1/4 cup sans sugar dim chocolate chips

Guidelines

1.   Line a heating sheet with material paper.

2.   Combine the margarine and sugar in an enormous bowl. Utilize a hand blender to beat until cushioned. Beat in the vanilla and molasses until very much consolidated.

3.   In a little bowl, mix together the almond flour, collagen powder, and ocean salt. Add the dry fixings to the enormous bowl. Beat with the hand blender until a brittle batter structure. Taste and alter sugar if necessary.

4.   Fold in the chocolate chips. Refrigerate for 20 minutes.

5.   Use a little cookie scoop to make little balls, about a tablespoon each, squeezing varying with your fingers. (You won't have the option to move them between your palms. Simply squeeze in the wake of discharging from the cookie scoop to make a uniform ball.) Place on the cookie sheet. Refrigerate for in any event 60 minutes, until firm.

Formula NOTES

Serving size: 2 1" nibbles

NUTRITION INFORMATION PER SERVING

Nutrition Facts

Sum per serving. Serving size in formula notes above.

Calories169

Fat14g

Protein9g

All out Carbs4g

Net Carbs3g

Fiber1g

Sugar1g

38. LEMON POPPY SEED LOW CARB KETO POUND CAKE RECIPE WITH ALMOND FLOUR

This simple lemon poppy seed bundt cake with almond flour has no sugar or grains. It's the best low carb keto pound cake formula I've at any point had - and prep takes only 15 minutes!

Course Breakfast, Dessert

.

Calories 248 kcal

Planning Time 15 minutes

Cook Time 60 minutes

Complete Time 1 hour 15 minutes

Servings

Fixings

Lemon Poppy Seed Bundt Cake

    3/4 cup Butter (mollified)

    1 cup Erythritol

    4 huge Egg (at room temperature)

    3/4 cup Sour cream

    2 tbsp Lemon extricate

    2 tsp Vanilla concentrate (discretionary)

    3 cup Blanched almond flour

    2 tsp sans gluten heating powder

    3 tbsp Poppy seeds

    1/2 tsp Sea salt

Lemon Glaze

    3/4 cup Powdered erythritol

    1/4 cup Lemon juice

    1/4 tsp Vanilla concentrate (discretionary)

Guidelines

1.   Preheat the broiler to 350 degrees F (177 degrees C). Oil a bundt skillet and put it in a safe spot.

2.   In an enormous, utilize a hand blender to beat together the margarine and sugar until cushioned.

3.   Beat in the eggs, acrid cream, lemon concentrate, and vanilla concentrate.

4.   In a new bowl, mix the almond flour preparing powder, poppy seeds, and ocean salt. Beat the dry fixings into the wet, about a cup at once.

5.   Transfer the hitter to the skillet and smooth the top. Heat for 40 min. or until the top is dim brilliant dark-colored. Spread freely with foil and keep preparing for 20-35 minutes, or until an embedded toothpick tells the truth. Let cool for at any rate 15 minutes in the skillet. At that point, turn out onto a cooling rack and cool totally.

6.   To make the coating, whisk together the powdered sugar, lemon juice, and vanilla concentrate—shower over the cake.

Formula NOTES

Serving size: 1 cut, or 1/16 of the whole formula

NUTRITION INFORMATION PER SERVING

Nutrition Facts

Sum per serving. Serving size in formula notes above.

Calories248

Fat23g

Protein7g

Complete Carbs6g

Net Carbs4g

Fiber2g

Sugar1g

39. LOW CARB KETO SUGAR-FREE CARROT CAKE RECIPE WITH ALMOND FLOUR

The best keto low carb carrot cake formula ever! The means for how to make sans sugar carrot cake are shockingly simple. So soggy and delightful, nobody will get it's without gluten and sans sugar. Paleo and sans dairy alternatives, as well.

Course Dessert

.

Calories 359 kcal

Planning Time 25 minutes

Cook Time 30 minutes

Complete Time 55 minutes

Servings cuts

This can't be played

Fixings

3/4 cup Erythritol (or coconut sugar for paleo)

3/4 cup Butter (relaxed; use coconut or ghee for paleo or without dairy)

1 tbsp Blackstrap molasses (discretionary)

1 tsp Vanilla concentrate

1/2 tsp Pineapple separate (discretionary)

4 enormous Egg

2 1/2 cup Blanched almond flour

2 tsp without gluten preparing powder

2 tsp Cinnamon

1/2 tsp Sea salt

2 1/2 cup Carrots (ground, estimated approximately stuffed in the wake of grinding)

1 1/2 cup Pecans (hacked; separated into 1 cup and 1/2 cup)

2 full recipes without sugar cream cheddar icing (twofold the icing formula; for paleo or sans dairy, overlook or utilize a coconut cream based icing)

Directions

1.   Preheat the cooker to 350 degrees F (177 degrees C). Line two 9 in (23 cm) round cake container with material paper. (Use springform skillet in the event that you have them.) Grease the base and sides.

2.   In a huge bowl, put together the margarine and erythritol until fleecy. Beat in the molasses (if utilizing), vanilla concentrate, and pineapple remove (if utilizing). Beat in the eggs, each in turn. Put in a safe spot.

3.   In another bowl, combine the almond flour, preparing powder, cinnamon, and ocean salt. Mix the dry fixings into the bowl with the wet fixings.

4.   Stir in the ground carrots. Overlay 1 cup (99 g) of the cleaved walnuts, holding the staying 1/2 cup (48.5 g).

5.   Transfer the hitter equally among the two arranged heating skillet. Heat for 30-35 minutes, until the top is springy.

6.   Let the cakes cool in the searches for gold minutes; at that point, move to a wire rack to cool totally.

7.   Meanwhile, make the without sugar icing as per the guidelines here. (Twofold the formula by entering "12" into the crate for # of servings on that page.)

8.   Ice, at that point, include the top layer and ice once more. Top with the staying cleaved walnuts.

Formula NOTES

Nutrition data incorporates the icing, in light of this sans sugar cream cheddar icing formula.

Serving size: 1 cut, or 1/16 of the whole formula

NUTRITION INFORMATION PER SERVING

Nutrition Facts

Sum per serving. Serving size in formula notes above.

Calories359

Fat34g

Protein7.5g

All out Carbs8.5g

Net Carbs5.5g

Fiber3g

Sugar2g

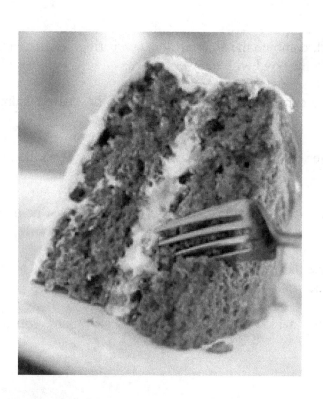

40. PINK HOMEMADE SUGAR-FREE GUMMY BEARS (RECIPE)

Need to realize how to make sticky holds on for only 3 fixings? It's simple! These pink without sugar sticky bears are made with genuine strawberries!

Course Snack

Calories 20 kcal

Planning Time 5 minutes

Cook Time 10 minutes

Absolute Time 15 minutes

Servings (10 little sticky bears for each serving)

Fixings

12 oz Strawberries (cut into quarters; equal to a 1 16 ounces compartment)

2/3 cup Water

1/3 cup Powdered erythritol (or somewhat more in the event that you need them better)

3 tbsp Vital Proteins Grass-Fed Gelatin

1/4 tsp Strawberry remove (discretionary, for more grounded strawberry, enhance)

Directions

1.   Place the strawberries and water into a pot. Stew over medium warmth, until the water turns red and strawberries extremely delicate (fairly soft) and pale in shading.

2.   Transfer the strawberries and fluid to a blender. Puree for some time until as smooth as could reasonably be expected.

3.   Wipe any pieces out of the pan. Empty the strawberry puree once again into the container.

(Discretionary adaptation: For the nearest surface to customary chewy candies, press the puree through a fine work strainer to get any seeds and a large portion of the mash. This takes some exertion and time, so you can without much of a stretch skip it and simply empty all the puree into the skillet.)

4. Add the powdered sugar to the dish. Warmth over medium-low warmth, mixing habitually, until the sugar breaks down. Try not to bubble. Taste and change sugar on the off chance that you need the final product better.

5. Reduce warmth to low. Mix in the strawberry extricates, if utilizing. Slowly sprinkle the gelatin into the dish, 1/2 or 1 tablespoon (7 to 14 g) at once, while whisking continually. Let the gelatin completely break up before including the following tablespoon. Keep racing until completely broken down.

6. Pour the fluid into molds, or into a material lined skillet (to cut later) on the off chance that you don't have molds. You can utilize a dropper in the event that you have only one.

7. Pop the sticky confirms of the molds, or cut in the event that you utilized a skillet. Put in the fridge or at room temperature.

Formula NOTES

As composed, these sans sticky sugar bears are not overly sweet. If you need them better, somewhat more sugar is fine to include.

Serving size: 10 sticky bears, or 1/10 of the whole formula

NUTRITION INFORMATION PER SERVING

Nutrition Facts

Sum per serving. Serving size in formula notes above.

Calories20

Fat0.1g

Protein3g

All out Carbs3g

Net Carbs2g

Fiber1g

Sugar2g

41. KETO LOW CARB PEANUT BUTTER OF PROTEIN BALLS RECIPE - 4 INGREDIENTS

These no heat low carb peanut spread protein balls with protein powder are fast and simple to make. Only 4 fixings and 10 minutes prep!

Course Breakfast, Snack

.

Calories 92 kcal

Planning Time 10 minutes

All out Time 30 minutes

Servings protein balls

Fixings

    1 cup Peanut margarine (thick and rich, salted)

    1/2 cup Dr. Hatchet KetoProtein Vanilla (~41g; or Dr. Hatchet Multi Collagen Protein Powder for form without stevia)

    1/2 cup Powdered erythritol (to taste)

    2 tsp Vanilla concentrate

    1/2 cup Peanuts (discretionary)

Directions

1.   Combine the peanut spread, protein powder, sugar, and vanilla in a ground-breaking blender or food processor. Heartbeat until uniform, scratching down the sides as vital. The blend ought to be thick, yet ready to be squeezed together. In the event that it's excessively slim, you can include more protein powder or potentially sugar to taste.

2.   Optional: Stir in the slashed peanuts, in the event that you like a little crunch. You can beat a few times in the event that it helps blend them in, however, don't completely process or they will discharge their oils and change the consistency of the peanut spread protein balls toward the end.

3.   Optional: Freeze the batter for around 20 minutes to make the blend firmer and less clingy.

4.   Use a little cookie scoop (or a spoon) to get chunks of batter. Fold into balls, ideally utilizing cold hands (wash them with cold water first). Keep refrigerated until prepared to eat.

Formula NOTES

Store the low carb peanut spread protein balls in the cooler, or freeze for more.

Serving size: 1 peanut jelly belly

NUTRITION INFORMATION PER SERVING

Nutrition Facts

Sum per serving. Serving size in formula notes above.

Calories92

Fat7.5g

Protein4g

Absolute Carbs3g

Net Carbs2g

Fiber1g

Sugar0.2g

42. LOW CARB KETO CREAM CHEESE OF COOKIES RECIPE - QUICK and EASY

These low carb keto cream cheddar cookies are so quick and simple to make! Only 6 fixings, 10 minutes prep, and 15 minutes in the stove.

Course Dessert

.

Calories 110 kcal

Planning Time 10 minutes

Cook Time 15 minutes

Absolute Time 25 minutes

Creator Maya Krampf from WholesomeYum.com

Servings 2" cookies

Fixings

1/4 cup Butter (mollified)

2 oz Cream cheddar (mollified)

1/3 cup of Besti Monk Fruit Allulose Blend (or up to 1/2 cup in the event that you like them sweet)

1 enormous Egg

2 tsp Vanilla concentrate

1/4 tsp Sea salt

1 tbsp Sour cream (discretionary)

3 cups Blanched almond flour

Guidelines

1. Preheat the broiler to 350 degrees F (177 degrees C). Line an enormous cookie sheet with material paper.

2. Use a hand blender or stand blender to beat together the margarine, cream cheddar, and sugar, until it's soft and light in shading.

3. Beat in the vanilla concentrate, salt, and egg. Beat in harsh cream, if utilizing (discretionary).

4. Beat the almond flour, 1/2 cup (64 g) at once. (The mixture will be thick and somewhat brittle, however, should stick when squeezed together.)

5. Use a medium cookie scoop (around 1/2 tbsp, 22 mL volume) to scoop bundles of the batter onto the readied cookie sheet. Smooth with your palm.

6. Bake for 15 min. till the edges are delicately brilliant. Permit to cool totally in the dish before taking care of (cookies will solidify as they cool).

Formula NOTES

Serving size: 1 2-inch cookie

Nutrition data does exclude discretionary acrid cream.

NUTRITION INFORMATION PER SERVING

Nutrition Facts

Sum per serving. Serving size in formula notes above.

Calories110

Fat10g

Protein3g

Complete Carbs3g

Net Carbs1g

Fiber2g

Sugar1g

43. THUMBPRINT CARAMEL PECAN TURTLE COOKIES RECIPE - GLUTEN FREE

An EASY caramel walnut turtle cookies formula that looks and tastes amazing! Nobody will accept these thumbprint cookies are without sugar and sans gluten.

Calories 170 kcal

Planning Time 20 minutes

Cook Time 12 minutes

All out Time 32 minutes

Servings cookies

Fixings

Sans gluten Shortbread Cookies

    2 1/2 cup Blanched almond flour

    6 tbsp Butter (relaxed)

    1/2 cup Erythritol

    1 tsp Vanilla concentrate

Filling and Topping

1/4 cup sans sugar caramel sauce

1/4 cup Pecans (18 walnut parts)

1/4 cup Nuts.com Sugar-Free Chocolate Chips (~1.5 oz)

1 tbsp Butter

Guidelines

1.   Make sans sugar caramel sauce as indicated by the directions here.

2.   Preheat the broiler to 350 degrees F (177 degrees C). Line a heating sheet with material paper.

3.   Make a shortbread cookie mixture as indicated by the directions here, yet don't prepare yet.

4.   Use a cookie scoop to put bundles of cookie mixture onto the heating sheet. Utilize the rear of a teaspoon size estimating spoon (or your thumb) to push down on each ball, creating a well in every cookie. A few breaks on the sides are alright, yet re-seal any enormous splits by squeezing together.

5.   Bake for 12-14 min. until the edges are brilliant. Cookies will be exceptionally delicate while they are hot - don't deal with. Cool for 10 minutes.

6.   While making an effort not to contact the cookie edges, utilize a little spoon to fill every cookie well with a teaspoon of caramel sauce. Press a walnut half on the caramel.

7.   Melt the chocolate chips and spread in the microwave or a twofold evaporator on the stove (mixing every so often). Sprinkle the chocolate over the cookies. Let the cookies cool totally before taking care of them.

Formula NOTES

Serving size: 1 cookie

NUTRITION INFORMATION PER SERVING

Nutrition Facts

Sum per serving. Serving size in formula notes above.

Calories170

Fat17g

Protein4g

All out Carbs5.5g

Net Carbs2g

Fiber3.5g

Sugar1g

44. SUGAR-FREE LOW CARB PEANUT BUTTER OF COOKIES RECIPE - 4 INGREDIENTS

Need to realize how to make natively constructed peanut margarine cookies without flour? You'll cherish this sans sugar low carb peanut margarine cookies formula. 4 fixings!!

Course Dessert

.

Calories 94 kcal

Planning Time 10 minutes

Cook Time 15 minutes

All out Time 25 minutes

Servings 2" cookies

Fixings

    1 1/4 cup Peanut margarine (smooth, salted)

    2 enormous Egg

    1/2 cup Erythritol (or any granulated sugar; utilize 1/3 cup for less sweet cookies)

    1 tsp Vanilla concentrate (discretionary)

    1/4 tsp of sea salt (1/2 tsp in the event that you like salty-sweet!)

    3/4 cup Peanuts (estimated entire and shelled, at that point coarsely hacked)

Directions

1.   Preheat the coo to 350 degrees F (177 degrees C). Line a preparing sheet with material paper.

2.   Place the peanut spread, egg, sugar, vanilla, and salt in a food processor. Procedure until smooth, scratching down the sides if necessary.

3.   Pulse in the peanut pieces until simply consolidated. (Don't overmix - you need a few pieces left for crunch.)

4.   Use a medium cookie scoop to put chunks of mixture onto the readied cookie sheet. Press the cookie batter into the scoop firmly before discharging onto the sheet. Smooth utilizing a fork in a bungle design. Between cookies, plunge the fork in a cup with cold water and afterward wipe with a paper towel. (This will forestall staying.)

5.   Bake for around 15-20 minutes until gently brilliant. Cool totally before taking care of. Cookies will get fresh as they cool.

Formula NOTES

Serving size: 1 2-inch cookie

NUTRITION INFORMATION PER SERVING

Nutrition Facts

Sum per serving. Serving size in formula notes above.

Calories94

Fat7g

Protein4g

Complete Carbs3g

Net Carbs2g

Fiber1g

Sugar0.2g

45. QEASY SUGAR-FREE LEMON MERINGUE COOKIES RECIPE - 4 INGREDIENTS

Perceive how to make meringue cookies that are healthy and delectable! These simple sans sugar lemon meringue cookies without cream of tartar need only 4 fixings.

Course Dessert

Food French

Calories 2 kcal

Planning Time 15 minutes

Cook Time 60 minutes

Absolute Time 3 hours 15 minutes

Servings (2 cookies each)

Fixings

2 huge Egg whites (at room temperature)

1/2 tsp Lemon juice

1/4 cup Powdered erythritol

1/2 tbsp Lemon pizzazz

Guidelines

1. Preheat the broiler to 200 degrees F (93 degrees C). Line an enormous preparing sheet with material paper.

2. Place the egg whites into an enormous bowl. Beat utilizing a hand blender at medium speed, until the whites get hazy and foamy.

3. Add the lemon juice. Speed up to high. Keep on beating until hardened pinnacles structure.

4. Gradually include the powdered sugar, a tablespoon at once, beating more as you go.

5. Gently overlap in the lemon pizzazz.

6. Carefully exchange the blend into a funneling pack. Channel cookies onto the lined heating sheet, about a teaspoon each, separated about an inch separated.

7. Bake for 1-2 hours. (Time will differ contingent upon the size and thickness of your meringues.) The meringues are done when they are firm and discharge effectively from the material paper, yet before they turn dark-colored. At the point when they are done, turn off the

stove and prop the entryway open with a wooden spoon. Leave the meringues in the stove along these lines for at any rate 60 minutes, until dry and fresh.

Formula NOTES

Serving size: 2 cookies

NUTRITION INFORMATION PER SERVING

Nutrition Facts

Sum per serving. Serving size in formula notes above.

Calories2

Fat0.01g

Protein0.3g

Complete Carbs0.04g

Net Carbs0.039g

Fiber0.001g

Sugar0.03g

46. LOW CARB PEANUT BUTTER CHOCOLATE NO BAKE COOKIES RECIPE

These low carb peanut spread chocolate no heat cookies are anything but difficult to make with only 5 fixings and taste stunning. The best no prepare cookies I've at any point attempted!

Course Dessert

.

Calories 123 kcal

Planning Time 10 minutes

All out Time 40 minutes

Servings 2" cookies

Fixings

1/2 cup of Powdered erythritol (or any powdered sugar, to taste)

3 tbsp Cocoa powder

2/3 cup Peanut margarine (rich, salted)

1/2 tsp Vanilla concentrate

1/2 cup Almonds (coarsely cleaved)

2 tbsp without sugar dull chocolate chips (discretionary)

Directions

1.   In a food processor, beat together the sugar and cocoa powder, until blended. Include the peanut spread and vanilla. Procedure until smooth and shiny. Change sugar to taste if necessary. (The batter will be extremely thick, yet should stick when squeezed together. In the event that it's fine or brittle, you may need to include progressively peanut spread, contingent upon how thick yours is.)

2.   Pulse in the almond pieces until simply joined. (Don't overmix - you need pieces for crunch.)

3.   Line a cookie sheet with material paper. Utilize a cookie scoop to scoop the mixture, press it in solidly, at that point discharge onto the cookie sheet. Utilize the palm of your hand to tenderly press down on every cookie ball to smooth. In the event that utilizing chocolate chips (discretionary), press them into the highest points of the cookies.

4.   Refrigerate for at any rate 30 minutes to solidify more. Store in the cooler.

Formula NOTES

Nutrition data does exclude discretionary chocolate chips.

Serving size: 1 2-inch cookie

NUTRITION INFORMATION PER SERVING

Nutrition Facts

Sum per serving. Serving size in formula notes above.

Calories123

Fat10g

Protein5g

All out Carbs5g

Net Carbs3g

Fiber2g

Sugar0.04g

47. THE CHOCOLATE-AVOCADO BROWNIES RECIPE

The most effortless, best chocolate avocado brownies formula - SUPER FUDGY! You'll never figure they are low carb, keto, without sugar, sans gluten, and even paleo.

Course Dessert

.

Calories 158 kcal

Planning Time 10 minutes

Cook Time 18 minutes

All out Time 28 minutes

Servings brownies

Fixings

1/2 cup butter

6 oz without sugar dull chocolate

1 medium Avocado

2 huge Egg (whisked delicately)

1 tsp Vanilla concentrate

1/2 cup of besti Monk Fruit Erythritol Blend (or any granulated sugar of decision)

3/4 cup Blanched almond flour

1/4 cup Cocoa powder (unsweetened)

Directions

1.
Preheat the stove to 325 degrees F (163 degrees C). Line a 9x9 in (23x23 cm) preparing skillet with foil or material paper and oil gently. Clasp the edges of the liner to the skillet with plastic clasps. (This is impermanent. They don't should be stove safe.) Set aside.

2.
Melt the spread and chocolate in a twofold evaporator on the stove. (Bubble water in a pot, place the spread and chocolate into a warmth evidence bowl, and spot on the pot. Warmth, mixing once in a while, until dissolved.) Set aside to cool for a few minutes.

3.   Put the avocado, the eggs, and vanilla in a powerful blender or food processor. Puree until smooth. Include the softened spread/chocolate blend and puree once more.

4.
In a littler bowl, mix together the almond flour, cocoa powder, and sugar. Add the dry fixings to the blender or food processor and mix in with a spatula. Heartbeat a couple of times until simply consolidated, scratching down the sides varying. (Don't overmix.)

5.
Spread the player into the readied heating skillet. It will be thick, so the clasps on the material or foil will help. Smooth the top with a spatula. Expel the clasps.

6.
Bake around 18-20 minutes, until brownies are scarcely set. The top should never again be wet, yet at the same time be delicate. An embedded toothpick will turn out with only a modest quantity of hitter on it. Cool totally to solidify before cutting.

Formula NOTES

Serving size: 1 brownie, or 1/16 of the skillet

I utilize this stevia improved sans sugar dull chocolate. It doesn't have a delayed flavor impression regardless of whether you don't care for stevia. In the event that you like to utilize totally unsweetened pastry specialist's chocolate, it should work, however you'll have to build the granulated sugar to taste.

NUTRITION INFORMATION PER SERVING

Nutrition Facts

Sum per serving. Serving size in formula notes above.

Calories158

Fat15g

Protein3g

All out Carbs9g

Net Carbs2g

Fiber7g

Sugar0.4g

48. Simple LOW CARB SALTED CARAMEL PIE RECIPE

Nobody will figure this simple salted walnut caramel pie is without gluten and sans sugar. With only a couple of fixings, it'll be the best low carb pie you've attempted!

Course Dessert

.

Calories 392 kcal

Planning Time 20 minutes

Cook Time 30 minutes

All out Time 50 minutes

Servings cuts

Fixings

1 formula Almond flour pie outside layer

3 recipes sans sugar caramel sauce (triple the formula, for 2 1/2 cup sauce absolute)

Sea salt (to taste)

1 cup Heavy cream

3 tbsp Powdered erythritol

1/2 tsp Vanilla concentrate

1/4 cup Pecans (discretionary; slashed, ideally toasted)

Guidelines

1.
Prepare the sans sugar caramel sauce as indicated by the guidelines here. Add ocean salt to taste toward the end. (You have to significantly increase the formula - simply enter 36 in the quantity of servings on the formula card. It will take more time to thicken when significantly increasing the formula - you'll have to stew the second step for in any event 30 minutes. A huge pot works best.)

2.
Meanwhile, set up the almond flour pie hull as per the directions here. Let the hull cool on the counter while you wrap up the caramel.

3.
Pour the caramel filling into the pie hull and smooth the top with a spatula. (Save 1/4 cup (32 g) caramel filling for fixing later.)

4.
Cool on the counter for 15 minutes. Spread with cling wrap, flush against the caramel surface. Refrigerate for in any event 2 hours, or medium-term, until firm. (You can refrigerate the saved 1/4 cup (32 g) for fixing in a different holder.)

5.
Using a hand blender, beat the overwhelming cream, powdered erythritol, and vanilla concentrate until firm pinnacles structure.

6.

Remove the cling wrap and spread the cream over the pie. Smooth the top with a spatula. If not serving immediately, refrigerate again until prepared to serve.

7.

Reheat the saved 1/4 cup (32 g) caramel in an extremely little pot over exceptionally low warmth, blending as often as possible, until it's pourable once more. Keep the warmth low to maintain a strategic distance from detachment or consuming. (In the event that it isolates, you might have the option to rescue it by whisking enthusiastically or utilizing a hand blender.) Drizzle over the pie. Top with hacked walnuts, if utilizing. Serve right away.

Formula NOTES

Discretionary walnuts excluded from nutrition data.

Serving size: 1 cut, or 1/16 of the pie

NUTRITION INFORMATION PER SERVING

Nutrition Facts

Sum per serving. Serving size in formula notes above.

Calories392

Fat40g

Protein5g

All out Carbs5g

Net Carbs3g

Fiber2g

Sugar2g

49. THE SUGAR-FREE KETO LOW-CARB & PEANUT BUTTER FUDGE RECIPE - 4 INGREDIENTS

This sans sugar keto low carb peanut margarine fudge formula is anything but difficult to make with only 4 fixings. Without gluten, with a sans dairy choice. So rich and velvety!

Course Dessert

Calories 189 kcal

Planning Time 5 minutes

Cook Time 5 minutes

All out Time 40 minutes

Servings (2x2" squares)

This can't be played in view of a specialized

Fixings

1 1/2 cup Peanut margarine (rich, salted)

    6 tbsp of Butter

2/3 cup of powdered erythritol (and any powdered sugar)

1/4 cup Dr. Hatchet Multi Collagen Protein Powder

1 tsp Vanilla concentrate (discretionary)

Directions

1.
Line a 8x8 in (20x20 cm) preparing skillet with material paper, letting it hang over the sides. Put in a safe spot.

2.
Combine the peanut spread and margarine in a huge bowl (if utilizing the microwave) or pot (if utilizing the stove). Warmth over low warmth, mixing a couple of times, until softened and smooth.

3.
Stir in the sugar and collagen powder, until smooth. Taste and alter sugar if necessary. Expel from heat. Mix in vanilla concentrate.

4.

Spread the blend into the heating container. Freeze for 30-45 minutes, until firm.

5.

To cut, lift the material paper out of the skillet and spot on a cutting board. Run a blade under high temp water to warm it up, dry, and use it to cut the fudge into squares. Store in the cooler. Whenever wanted, mellow on the counter for two or three minutes when serving.

Formula NOTES

This without sugar peanut spread fudge is very filling. If you need to appreciate it as a reduced down treat with less carbs and calories, simply cut it into littler squares.

Serving size: 1 2x2" square

NUTRITION INFORMATION PER SERVING

Nutrition Facts

Sum per serving. Serving size in formula notes above.

Calories189

Fat16g

Protein8g

All out Carbs5g

Net Carbs3g

Fiber2g

Sugar0.04g

50. HEALTHY-CHOCOLATE PEANUT & BUTTER BARS RECIPE - THE GLUTEN FREE

These simple, healthy chocolate peanut margarine bars are the best mix of sans gluten shortbread outside, peanut spread and chocolate. 15 minutes prep!

Course Dessert

.

Calories 212 kcal

Planning Time 15 minutes

Cook Time 10 minutes

All out Time 25 minutes

Servings bars

Fixings

Shortbread Cookie Layer

1 cup Blanched almond flour

1/4 cup Besti Monk Fruit Erythritol Blend(or any granulated sweetener*)

3 tbsp Coconut oil

1/2 tsp Vanilla concentrate (discretionary)

Peanut Butter Layer

1/3 cup Powdered erythritol (or any powdered sweetener*)

1/3 cup Peanut flour (likewise called "peanut margarine powder"; ideally unsweetened**)

3/4 cup Peanut margarine (velvety, unsweetened***)

1/2 tsp Vanilla concentrate (discretionary)

Chocolate Layer

6 oz sans sugar dim chocolate

3 tbsp Coconut oil

1 tbsp Powdered erythritol (or any powdered sweetener*)

Directions

Cookie Layer

1. Preheat the cooker to 350 degrees F (177 degrees C). Line a 9x9 in (23x23 cm) heating skillet with material paper.

2. Mix the almond flour together and sugar.

3.
In a little bowl, mix together the dissolved coconut oil and vanilla. Blend into the almond flour blend, squeezing with the rear of a spoon or spatula, until a brittle mixture structures.

4.
Press the cookie mixture into the lined container. Heat for around 10 minutes, until the edges are brilliant. Cool for a couple of moments, until the top is firm and the container is sufficiently cool to deal with. (Then, make the peanut margarine layer.)

Peanut Butter Layer

1.mix together the peanut flour and sugar.

2.
Add the peanut margarine and vanilla. Blend well, squeezing with the rear of a spoon or spatula, until completely joined. (The blend will be thick and can require some push to consolidate. If you have an amazing blender or food processor, you can blend in there, scratching down the sides periodically.)

3.
Spoon bits of the peanut margarine mixture on the cookie layer in the skillet, at that point spread and press uniformly. On the off chance that it's clingy, working with wet hands can help (however not very wet to abstain from adding water to the peanut margarine blend).

Chocolate Layer

1.
Combine chocolate chips and coconut oil in a medium bowl. Warmth in the microwave (or on the stove in a twofold grill), blending at regular intervals, until totally liquefied.

2.
Whisk in the sugar.

3.

Pour the chocolate over the peanut margarine layer and spread equitably. Cool totally, until the chocolate is strong, before cutting into bars. (You can likewise refrigerate to speed the cooling procedure. Cut straight down with an enormous culinary specialist's blade (don't saw to and fro). When cut, refrigerate to store.

Formula NOTES

- In the shortbread cookie layer, you can utilize either a granulated or powdered sugar. In the peanut spread and chocolate layers, a powdered sugar is prescribed for a smooth surface. You may make your own powdered sugar by pounding granulated sugar through a food processor. Else, you can purchase the powdered erythritol I utilized here.

- Peanut flour and peanut margarine powder are the equivalent. Most markets convey peanut spread powder with a modest quantity of sugar - this is alright to utilize in case you're fine with that, however you'll likely need to diminish the sugar a bit. You can purchase peanut flour with no sugar included here.

- It's your decision in the event that you need to utilize salted or unsalted peanut spread, in the event that you need your bars to be somewhat salty or not. I loved them with daintily salted peanut margarine.

Serving size: 1 bar, or 1/16 of whole formula

NUTRITION INFORMATION PER SERVING

Nutrition Facts

Sum per serving. Serving size in formula notes above.

Calories212

Fat19g

Protein6g

Absolute Carbs11g

Net Carbs4g

Fiber7g

Sugar0.4g

51. SUGAR-FREE GLUTEN-FREE GRAHAM CRACKERS RECIPE

These natively constructed sans sugar sans gluten graham wafers with almond flour are speedy and simple. Heavenly as a tidbit or to make s'mores!

Course Snack

.

Calories 147 kcal

Planning Time 20 minutes

Cook Time 10 minutes

All out Time 30 minutes

Servings (2 3x3" saltines each)

Fixings

2 1/2 cup Blanched almond flour

1/2 cup Erythritol (or any sugar)

1/2 tbsp Cinnamon

1/2 tsp Sea salt

1 huge Egg

1 tbsp Butter (liquefied; use coconut oil for sans dairy)

1 tsp Vanilla concentrate

1 tsp Blackstrap molasses

1/4 tsp Honey concentrate (discretionary, for progressively valid flavor)

Guidelines

1.
Preheat the broiler to 350 degrees F (177 degrees C). Line a heating sheet with material paper.

2.
Combine the almond flour, sugar, cinnamon and ocean salt in a food processor. Heartbeat until combined, blending in from the sides varying.

3.   In a little bowl, whisk the eggs, margarine, vanilla, molasses, and nectar remove. Add to the food processor and procedure until a thick, clingy batter structures. Stop to scratch down the sides varying.

4.
When the mixture is uniform, expel from the food processor and structure into a ball. Freeze for around 10 minutes, until no longer clingy, or refrigerate until prepared to make saltines.

5.
Place the mixture ball between two enormous bits of material paper. Utilize a turning pin to turn out to square shape, around 1/16 to 1/8 in (1.5 to 3 cm) thick.

6.
Cut the wafer batter into squares. Cautiously strip the squares off the material and spot onto the lined heating sheet, without contacting. Prick gaps with a toothpick or fork. You'll have lopsided batter staying at the edges, so simply press that once more into a ball, turn out once more, and rehash. (You may require two heating sheets or two groups, contingent upon the size of your preparing sheet.)

7.
Bake for 8-12 minutes, until brilliant. Cool totally until firm.

Formula NOTES

Number of wafers is surmised, on the grounds that it relies upon how meagerly you reveal the batter. A serving is 1/12 of the whole formula.

Serving size: 2 3x3" wafers

NUTRITION INFORMATION PER SERVING

Nutrition Facts

Sum per serving. Serving size in formula notes above.

Calories147

Fat12g

Protein6g

Absolute Carbs6g

Net Carbs3g

Fiber3g

Sugar1g

52. SUGAR-FREE MARSHMALLOWS RECIPE WITHOUT CORN SYRUP

You just need 4 fixings to make custom made sans sugar marshmallows, no corn syrup required!

Course Dessert

.

Calories 6 kcal

Planning Time 15 minutes

Cook Time 5 minutes

All out Time 20 minutes

Servings

Fixings

2 tbsp Unflavored gelatin powder

1 cup Water (warm, partitioned)

1 1/2 cups Besti Powdered Monk Fruit Allulose Blend

1/4 tsp Sea salt

2 tsp Vanilla concentrate

Guidelines

1.
Line a 8x8 in (20x20 cm) container with material paper. Put in a safe spot.

2.
Pour 1/2 cup (118 mL) warm water into an enormous bowl (it will scarcely cover the base of the bowl). Sprinkle gelatin over the water and whisk right away. Put in a safe spot.

3.
Meanwhile, include staying 1/2 cup (118 mL) water, powdered sugar, and ocean salt to an enormous pan. Warmth over low to medium warmth for a couple of moments, mixing as often as possible, until the blend is hot, however not bubbling, and sugar breaks down. (The shading will change from murky to somewhat translucent, and evacuate quickly when you see bubbles beginning to frame at the edges.)

4.
Remove from heat. Mix in vanilla concentrate. Empty the hot fluid into the huge bowl with gelatin, while whisking continually.

5.
Using a hand blender on high force, beat the blend for around 12-15 minutes, until the volume duplicates and the blend looks feathery, similar to solid egg white pinnacles. (The time could take longer relying upon the size of your bowl and how ground-breaking your blender is.)

6.
Transfer the marshmallow blend into the readied skillet.

7.
Refrigerate for at any rate 8 hours, or medium-term, until firm and no longer clingy. Utilize a sharp gourmet expert's blade to cut into squares.

Formula NOTES

Serving size: 4 1-inch marshmallows each

This formula was refreshed in December 2019 to utilize the new Besti Monk Fruit Allulose Blend. The past rendition utilized a similar measure of powdered erythritol joined with 1/2 teaspoon vanilla stevia. You can at present make the old rendition, however, I found that the priest organic product allulose mix is way better - the surface is practically indistinguishable from genuine marshmallows made with sugar!

NUTRITION INFORMATION PER SERVING

Nutrition Facts

Sum per serving. Serving size in formula notes above.

Calories6

Fat0g

Protein1g

Absolute Carbs0.1g

Net Carbs0.1g

Fiber0g

Sugar0.1g

53. Simple KETO LOW CARB PUMPKIN PIE RECIPE (SUGAR-FREE, GLUTEN-FREE)

You just need a couple of elements for this simple keto low carb pumpkin pie formula with almond flour covering. It will be your preferred without sugar pumpkin pie!

Course Dessert

.

Calories 244 kcal

Planning Time 15 minutes

Cook Time 45 minutes

All out Time 60 minutes

Servings cuts

Fixings

1 formula Almond flour pie covering (or your preferred pie outside layer formula)

1 15-oz would pumpkin be able to puree

1/2 cup of heavy cream (or coconut cream for sans dairy/paleo)

2 enormous Egg (at room temperature)

2/3 cup Powdered erythritol

2 tsp Pumpkin pie zest

1/4 tsp Sea salt

1 tsp Vanilla concentrate (discretionary)

1 tsp Blackstrap molasses (discretionary)

Guidelines

1.
Make the sweet almond flour pie outside layer as per the headings here.

2.
Meanwhile, beat together all outstanding fixings at medium-low speed, until smooth. (Don't overmix.)

3.
When the pie hull is finished preparing, diminish the stove temperature to 325 degrees F (163 degrees C). Cool the outside layer on the counter for in any event 10 minutes, longer on the off chance that you have time.

4.
Pour the filling into the hull. Tenderly tap on the counter to discharge air bubbles.

5.   Bake it for 40-50 min., until the pie, is nearly set yet somewhat jiggly in the inside. (Keep an eye on it once in a while, and in the event that you see the outside begin to dark-colored, spread

the covering edge with foil and come back to the stove until the filling is finished. It should even now shake a piece in the inside, similar to a custard before it sets.)

6.
Cool totally on the counter, at that point, refrigerate at any rate an hour prior to cutting. Pie can be refrigerated medium-term.

Formula NOTES

To lessen the opportunity of breaking your low carb pumpkin pie, you can prepare the pie in a water shower. Something else, in the event that you end up with splits, you can generally cover them with whipped cream.

Serving size: 1 cut, or 1/12 of the whole pie

NUTRITION INFORMATION PER SERVING

Nutrition Facts

Sum per serving. Serving size in formula notes above.

Calories244

Fat21g

Protein7g

Complete Carbs8g

Net Carbs4g

Fiber4g

Sugar2g

54. SUGAR-FREE KETO & PEANUT BUTTER CUPS RECIPES - 5 INGREDIENTS

These without sugar keto peanut spread cups are much the same as genuine ones! You'll adore this simple low carb peanut margarine cup formula made with 5 fixings.

Course Dessert, Snack

.

Calories 187 kcal

Planning Time 10 minutes

Cook Time 5 minutes

All out Time 1 hour 5 minutes

Servings peanut margarine cups

Fixings

Chocolate layers

10 oz without sugar dim chocolate (separated; see notes on the chocolate to utilize, don't utilize pastry specialist's chocolate!)

5 tbsp Coconut oil (separated)

1/2 tsp Vanilla concentrate (discretionary, separated)

Peanut spread layer

3 1/2 tbsp Peanut spread (velvety)

2 tsp Coconut oil

4 tsp Powdered erythritol (to taste)

1 1/2 tsp Peanut flour

1/8 tsp Vanilla concentrate (discretionary)

1 squeeze Sea salt (discretionary, to taste)

Directions

1.　　Line a biscuit dish with material paper liners (or candy cups).

2.　　For the base chocolate layer, heat and melt half of the chocolate to 5 oz, or 142 g and also, half of the coconut oil (2 1/2 tbsp, 35 g) in a twofold evaporator on the stove, blending much of the time, until softened. (You can likewise warm in the microwave, blending at 20 second interims.)

3.
Fill the base of the material cups uniformly with chocolate (around 2 tsp (10 mL) in each). Freeze for 10 minutes, until in any event the top is firm.

4.　　Meanwhile, for the peanut margarine layer, heat the peanut spread and coconut oil in a twofold kettle or microwave (same strategy as stage 2). Mix in the powdered sugar, peanut flour, vanilla (if utilizing), and ocean salt (if utilizing), until smooth. Alter sugar and salt to taste whenever wanted.

5.
Spoon a teaspoon of the peanut margarine blend onto the focal point of each cup over the chocolate layer. Freeze for an additional 10 minutes, until in any event the top is firm.

6.　　Meanwhile, make the top chocolate layer. Warmth the rest of the chocolate (5 oz, 142 g) and remaining coconut oil (2 1/2 tbsp, 35 g) in a twofold kettle or microwave (same strategy as stage 2). Mix in the staying vanilla (1/4 tsp, 1 mL), if utilizing.

7.　　Pour the melt chocolate into the cups, over the peanut margarine layer (around 2 tsp (10 mL) in each). The chocolate will occupy the unfilled space on the sides of the peanut margarine circles and furthermore spread the top.

8.
Return to the cooler for in any event 20-30 minutes, until totally firm. Store in the cooler.

Formula NOTES

Significant: You need without sugar dull chocolate like this, not unsweetened preparing chocolate.

Serving size: 1 piece

NUTRITION INFORMATION PER SERVING

Nutrition Facts

Sum per serving. Serving size in formula notes above.

Calories187

Fat18g

Protein3g

Complete Carbs14g

Net Carbs3g

Fiber11g

Sugar0.1g

55. HEALTHY PUMPKIN MUFFINS RECIPE WITH COCONUT FLOUR and ALMOND FLOUR

This low carb pumpkin biscuits formula with coconut flour and almond flour is overly sodden and EASY! You can likewise make these keto pumpkin biscuits paleo or without nut in the event that you'd like.

Course Breakfast, Snack

.

Calories 173 kcal

Planning Time 10 minutes

Cook Time 25 minutes

All out Time 35 minutes

Servings biscuits

Fixings

1/2 cup of coconut flour

1/2 cup of blanched almond flour (or sunflower seed meal*)

1/2 cup of Allulose (or any sugar of decision)

1 tbsp without gluten preparing powder

1 tbsp Pumpkin pie flavor

1/4 tsp Sea salt

4 huge Eggs

3/4 cup pumpkin puree

1/2 cup Ghee (estimated strong, at that point liquefied; can sub spread or coconut oil)

1 tsp Vanilla concentrate

Pumpkin seeds (for fixing - discretionary)

Directions

1.   Preheat the cooker to 350 degrees F (177 degrees C). Line 10 biscuit cups with material liners.

2.   In a huge bowl, mix together the coconut flour, almond flour, sugar, preparing powder, pumpkin pie zest, and ocean salt. Ensure there are no clusters.

3.   Stir in the eggs, pumpkin puree, liquefied ghee, and vanilla, until totally consolidated.

4.   Spoon the hitter uniformly into the biscuit cups and smooth the tops. (They ought to be practically full, not 2/3 or 3/4 full.) If wanted, sprinkle pumpkin seeds on top and press delicately.

5.   Bake for around 25 minutes, until an embedded toothpick tells the truth, and the biscuits are marginally brilliant around the edges.

Formula NOTES

Serving size: 1 biscuit

- Sunflower seed meal will work for a without nut variant. Nutrition data depends on almond flour.

-

This formula was refreshed on 09/28/2018 to make increasingly soggy biscuits. The first form had 1/3 cup ghee and 1/2 cup pumpkin puree. Photographs show the refreshed form.

-

This formula initially utilized erythritol and was refreshed on 12/30/2019 to utilize allulose. This helps make the low carb pumpkin biscuits significantly increasingly wet and delicate; however you can even now utilize erythritol in the event that you like. The sugar sum was likewise decreased from 2/3 cup sugar to 1/2 cup, in light of peruser input.

NUTRITION INFORMATION PER SERVING

Nutrition Facts

Sum per serving. Serving size in formula notes above.

Calories173

Fat14g

Protein4g

All out Carbs7g

Net Carbs4g

Fiber3g

Sugar1g

56. LOW CARB DONUTS RECIPE - ALMOND FLOUR KETO DONUTS (PALEO, GLUTEN FREE)

This low carb doughnuts formula with almond flour is anything but difficult to make. These keto doughnuts taste simply like standard glossed over ones, with alternatives for paleo doughnuts, as well!

Course Breakfast, Dessert

-

Calories 257 kcal

Planning Time 15 minutes

Cook Time 25 minutes

All out Time 40 minutes

Servings doughnuts

Fixings

Doughnuts

1 cup Blanched almond flour

1/4 cup Besti Monk Fruit Erythritol Blend

2 tsp sans gluten preparing powder

1 tsp Cinnamon

1/8 tsp Sea salt

1/4 cup Butter (unsalted; estimated strong, at that point softened)

1/4 cup unsweetened almond milk

2 enormous Egg

1/2 tsp Vanilla concentrate

Cinnamon Coating

1/2 cup Besti Monk Fruit Erythritol Blend

1 tsp Cinnamon

3 tbsp Butter (unsalted; estimated strong, at that point softened)

Guidelines

1.
Preheat the broiler to 350 degrees F (177 degrees C). Oil a doughnut dish well.

2.
In an enormous bowl, mix together the almond flour, sugar, preparing powder, cinnamon, and ocean salt.

3.
In a little bowl, whisk together the softened spread, almond milk, egg, and vanilla concentrate. Whisk the wet blend into the dry blend.

4.
Transfer the player equally into the doughnut holes, filling them 3/4 of the way. Prepare for around 22-28 minutes (or longer for a silicone skillet!), until dull brilliant dark-colored. Cool until doughnuts are anything but difficult to expel from the container.

5.
Meanwhile, in a little bowl, mix together the sugar and cinnamon for the covering.

6.
When the doughnuts have cooled enough to handily expel from the molds, move them to a cutting board. Brush the two sides of one doughnut with spread, at that point press/move in the sugar/cinnamon blend to cover. Rehash with the rest of the doughnuts.

Formula NOTES

Serving size: 1 doughnut

•
See extra tips for keto paleo doughnuts in the post above!

NUTRITION INFORMATION PER SERVING

Nutrition Facts

Sum per serving. Serving size in formula notes above.

Calories257

Fat25g

Protein6g

All out Carbs5g

Net Carbs3g

Fiber2g

Sugar1g

57. CHEESECAKE-COOKIES RECIPE

These simple raspberry cheesecake thumbprint cookies are sans gluten and low carb. A cream cheddar shortbread cookie with a raspberry whirl cheesecake focus!

Course Dessert

.

Calories 147 kcal

Planning Time 30 minutes

Cook Time 15 minutes

Complete Time 45 minutes

Servings 2-1/4" cookies

Fixings

Raspberry filling

1/2 bundle Driscoll's Raspberries (3 ounces or ~2/3 cup)

1 1/2 tbsp Powdered erythritol

Cream cheddar filling

4 oz Cream cheddar (mellowed)

2 tbsp Powdered erythritol

1/2 tsp Vanilla concentrate

1/2 enormous Egg (whisk an entire egg and utilize 1/2 of that or around 1/2 tablespoons)

Cookies

1/4 cup Butter (mellowed)

1 oz Cream cheddar (mellowed)

1/2 cup Erythritol

1/2 enormous Egg (utilize remaining whisked egg from filling)

1 tsp Vanilla concentrate

2 1/2 cup Blanched almond flour

Guidelines

Raspberry filling

1.
Puree the raspberries and powdered erythritol in a blender. Press fluid through a fine work sifter over a little pot. Dispose of seeds trapped in the sifter.

2.

Bring the raspberry sauce to a delicate stew. Stew the raspberry sauce delicately over low warmth for around 3-5 minutes, until the volume is diminished by around 1/3. Expel from warmth and permit to cool to room temperature.

Cream cheddar filling

1.
Meanwhile, make the cream cheddar blend. Utilizing a hand blender or stand blender, beat the cream cheddar, powdered erythritol, and egg together until smooth. Beat in vanilla.

Cookies Assembly

1.   Preheat the cooker to 350 degrees F (177 degrees C). Line an enormous cookie sheet with material paper.

2.   Use a hand blender or stand blender to beat together the spread, cream cheddar, and erythritol, until it's feathery and light in shading.

3.   Beat in the vanilla concentrate and remaining egg.

4.   Beat the almond flour, 1/2 cup (64 g) at once. (The mixture will be thick and somewhat brittle, yet should stick when squeezed together.)

5.   Use a medium cookie scoop (around 2 tbsp (30 mL) volume) to scoop wads of the mixture onto the readied cookie sheet. (While scooping, level the batter level against the scoop.) Use the rear of a round teaspoon-size estimating spoon to push on the focal point of every mixture ball and make a huge well in the focal point of every cookie, smoothing all the while. In the event that any huge splits structure on the sides, press them back together (some littler breaks are fine to leave in its present condition).

6.   Use a little spoon to dab the cream cheddar blend into each well, filling yet not exactly full.

7.   Use a little spoon to spot littler measures of the diminished raspberry puree onto the focal point of every cookie. Utilize a toothpick to whirl into the cream cheddar.

8.   Bake for 10-12 min., till the edges are brilliant and filling is scarcely set. Permit to cool totally in the dish before taking care of (cookies will solidify as they cool).

Formula NOTES

Net carbs per serving (1 cookie): 3g

*Time sparing tip: For the prettiest and most uniform outcomes, utilize the technique above. Be that as it may, on the off chance that you'd prefer to make these all the more rapidly, you can whirl the cream cheddar blend and raspberry puree preceding adding to the cookies. Simply be mindful so as not to overmix - you need them twirled, not completely joined.

NUTRITION INFORMATION PER SERVING

Nutrition Facts

Sum per serving. Serving size in formula notes above.

Calories147

Fat13g

Protein4g

Complete Carbs5g

Net Carbs3g

Fiber2g

Sugar1g

58. LOW-CARB & PALEO ALMOND FLOUR PIE CRUST RECIPE - 5 INGREDIENTS

This low carb paleo almond flour pie hull formula is so natural to make. Only 5 minutes prep and 5 fixings! Without gluten, sans sugar, and keto.

Course Breakfast, Dessert, Main Course

.

Calories 180 kcal

Planning Time 5 minutes

Cook Time 10 minutes

Complete Time 15 minutes

Servings cuts

Fixings

2 1/2 cup Blanched almond flour

1/3 cup Erythritol (or any sugar of choice*; discard for exquisite pie covering)

1/4 tsp of Sea salt (or 1/2 tsp for exquisite pie outside layer)

1/4 cup Ghee (estimated strong, at that point softened)

1 enormous Egg (or ~2 tbsp extra ghee)

1/2 tsp Vanilla concentrate (discretionary)

Guidelines

1.
Preheat the broiler to 350 degrees F (177 degrees C). Line the base of a 9 in (23 cm) round pie skillet with material paper, or oil well.

2.   In an enormous bowl, combine the almond flour, erythritol (if utilizing), and ocean salt.

3.
Stir in the dissolved ghee and egg, until all around joined. (In the case of utilizing vanilla, mix that into the liquefied ghee before adding to the dry fixings.) The "batter" will be dry and brittle. Simply continue blending, squeezing and mixing, until it's uniform, and there is no almond flour powder left. (Then again, you can utilize a food processor to combine everything.)

4.
Press the mixture into the base of the readied skillet. You can woodwind the edges of wanted; on the off chance that it disintegrates while doing this, simply press it back together. Cautiously jab gaps in the surface utilizing a fork to forestall percolating.

5.   Bake for 10-12 minutes, until softly brilliant. (Include fillings simply after pre-heating.)

Formula NOTES

Sugar note: The measure of sugar that is best will fluctuate dependent on the filling. Utilize 1/3 cup for a sweet hull, 1/4 cup for a gently sweet outside (if your filling is excessively sweet), 1/2 cup for a sweet covering (on the off chance that you like a better outside layer or your filling is tart), OR discard sugar for the appetizing hull.

Serving size: 1 cut, or 1/12 of the whole formula

NUTRITION INFORMATION PER SERVING

Nutrition Facts

Sum per serving. Serving size in formula notes above.

Calories180

Fat17g

Protein6g

Absolute Carbs5g

Net Carbs2g

Fiber3g

Sugar1g

59. STRAWBERRY LEMONADE CAKE RECIPE (LOW CARB, GLUTEN-FREE, SUGAR-FREE)

This simple handcrafted strawberry lemonade cake formula needs 20 minutes planning time and 10 fixings. Nobody will get its low carb, sans sugar, and sans gluten!

Course Dessert

.

Calories 308 kcal

Planning Time 20 minutes

Cook Time 20 minutes

Complete Time 1 hour 40 minutes

Servings cuts

Fixings

Cake

1 1/3 cup Erythritol

3/4 cup Butter (mollified)

8 huge Egg

1/3 cup Sour cream

3 tbsp Lemon juice

2 tbsp Lemon pizzazz (discretionary, however, prescribed)

3 cup Blanched almond flour

1/2 cup Coconut flour

1 1/2 tbsp sans gluten heating powder

1/2 tsp Sea salt

1 1/4 cup Strawberries (cut meagerly)

Icing

1/2 cup Strawberries

1 1/2 cup Powdered erythritol

2/3 cup Sour cream

1 tbsp Lemon juice

1 cup Heavy cream

Directions

Strawberry Lemonade Cake

1.   Preheat the cooker to 350 degrees F (177 degrees C). Line the bottoms of two 9 in (23 cm) round springform dish with material paper.

2.
In a huge bowl, utilize a hand blender to beat together the spread and erythritol, until light in shading and somewhat soft.

3.
Beat in the eggs, each in turn, at that point the harsh cream, lemon juice, and lemon get-up-and-go.

4.
Beat in the almond flour, coconut flour, heating powder, and ocean salt.

5.
Transfer the player to the fixed skillet and smooth the top with a spatula. Prepare for 20-25 minutes, until the top is brilliant, and an embedded toothpick tells the truth.

Whipped Cream Frosting

1.
Puree the strawberries in a blender. Include the powdered erythritol, harsh cream, and lemon juice. Puree again until smooth.

2.
In a huge bowl, utilize a hand blender to beat overwhelming cream until solid pinnacles structure.

3.
Gradually crease in the strawberry blend, 1/4 to 1/2 cup (60 to 120 mL) at once, being mindful so as not to separate the whipped cream.

Get together

1.
Let the cake layers cool independently to room temperature.

2.
Frost the base cake layer first. Mastermind cut strawberries over the icing, at that point top with the subsequent cake layer. Refrigerate for in any event 60 minutes.

Formula NOTES

Serving size: 1 cut, or 1/16 of the whole cake

NUTRITION INFORMATION PER SERVING

Nutrition Facts

Sum per serving. Serving size in formula notes above.

Calories308

Fat28g

Protein9g

All out Carbs10g

Net Carbs5g

Fiber5g

Sugar3g

60. RASPBERRY ICE CREAM RECIPE - 3 INGREDIENTS, 2 MINUTES (LOW CARB, SUGAR-FREE, GLUTEN-FREE)

This simple raspberry dessert formula takes only 2 minutes and requires 3 fixings! It's a healthy method to fulfill your frozen yogurt needing right away.

Course Dessert

.

Calories 183 kcal

Planning Time 5 minutes

Absolute Time 5 minutes

Servings 1/2-cup servings

Fixings

1 cup Heavy cream (or coconut cream)

2 cup frozen raspberries

1/3 cup Powdered erythritol (or any sugar - to taste)

Directions

1.
Pour the cream into a blender. Mix until hardened pinnacles structure (you can likewise utilize a hand blender if your blender isn't ground-breaking enough to whip the cream).

2.
Add the solidified raspberries and sugar to the blender. Puree until consolidated. Change sugar to taste if necessary, and provided that this is true, puree once more.

3.
Optional: This frozen yogurt is a delicate serve consistency. If you lean toward a firmer frozen yogurt, you can run the blend through a dessert creator, or spot in the cooler to solidify. In the case of utilizing the cooler, mix each 30-an hour for the primary couple hours to separate any precious ice stones.

Formula NOTES

Serving size: 1/2 cup

NUTRITION INFORMATION PER SERVING

Nutrition Facts

Sum per serving. Serving size in formula notes above.

Calories183

Fat16g

Protein1g

Complete Carbs6g

Net Carbs3g

Fiber3g

Sugar2g

WATERMELON PIZZA RECIPE & CREAM CHEESE ICING (SUGAR-FREE, THE LOW CARB, GLUTEN-FREE)

This snappy and simple watermelon pizza formula with berries and cream cheddar icing makes an ideal healthy summer dessert. Prepared quickly!

Course Dessert

.

Calories 70 kcal

Planning Time 10 minutes

Absolute Time 10 minutes

Servings cuts

Fixings

3 tbsp Cream cheddar (mellowed, cut into 3D shapes)

3 tbsp Heavy cream

2 tbsp Powdered erythritol (or any powdered or fluid sugar; change in accordance with taste)

4 tsp Lemon juice

1/2 tsp Vanilla concentrate

1 round cut Watermelon (1" thick)

1/2 cup Blueberries

1/2 cup Raspberries

Guidelines

1.
Blend the cream cheddar, cream, powdered sugar, lemon juice, and vanilla in a blender until smooth. Alter sugar to taste.

2.
Drizzle, spread, or funnel the cream blend over the watermelon cut. Top with berries. Cut into 8 cuts.

Formula NOTES

Serving size: 1 cut, or 1/8 of the whole pizza

NUTRITION INFORMATION PER SERVING

Nutrition Facts

Sum per serving. Serving size in formula notes above.

Calories70

Fat4g

Protein1g

Complete Carbs8g

Net Carbs7g

Fiber1g

Sugar6g

CPSIA information can be obtained
at www.ICGtesting.com
Printed in the USA
BVHW050003280421
605946BV00004B/740